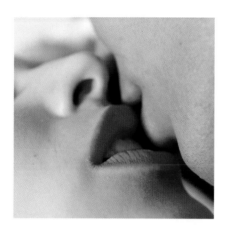

THE BEST-EVER ILLUSTRATED

SEX HANDBOOK

SUCCESSFUL TECHNIQUES AND NEW IDEAS FOR LONG-TERM LOVERS

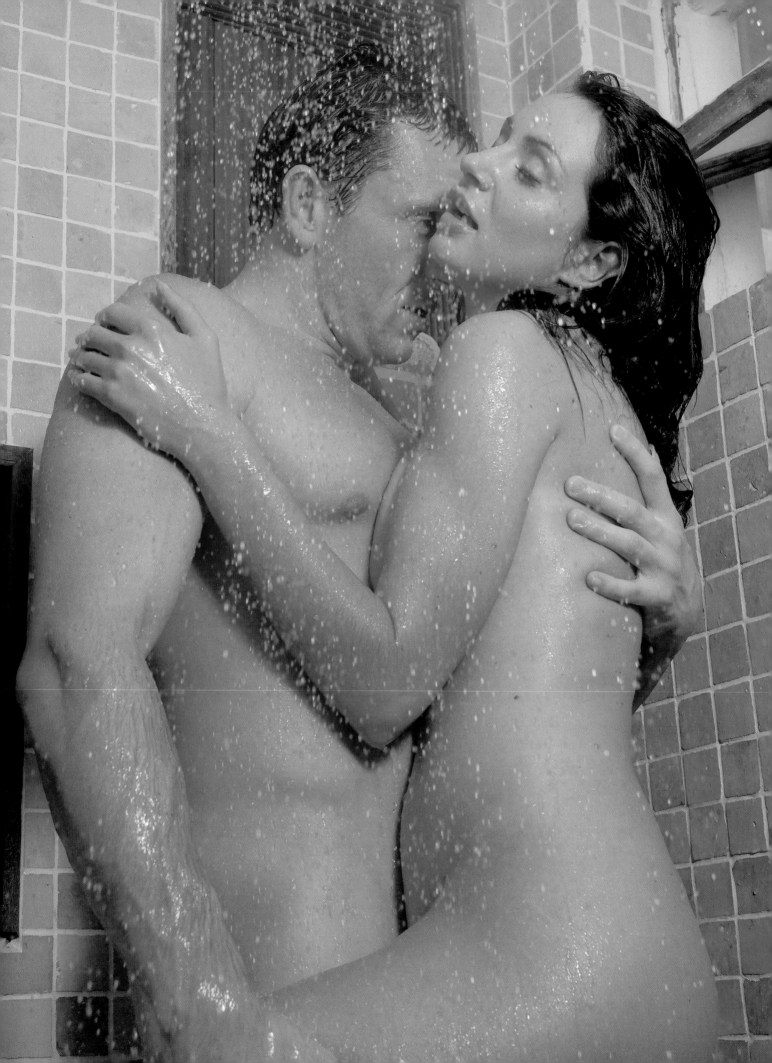

THE BEST-EVER ILLUSTRATED
SEX HANDBOOK

SUCCESSFUL TECHNIQUES AND NEW IDEAS FOR LONG-TERM LOVERS

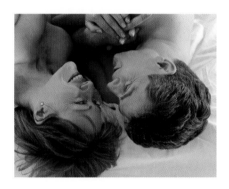

CONTAINS MORE THAN 200 BEAUTIFUL PHOTOGRAPHS INCLUDING STEP-BY-STEP SEQUENCES
TO DEMONSTRATE EVERYTHING FROM THE BASICS TO MORE ADVANCED POSITIONS

JUDY BASTYRA
PHOTOGRAPHY BY JOHN FREEMAN

HERMES
HOUSE

This edition is published by Hermes House, an imprint of Anness Publishing Ltd,
Hermes House, 88–89 Blackfriars Road, London SE1 8HA; tel. 020 7401 2077;
fax 020 7633 9499; www.hermeshouse.com; www.annesspublishing.com

If you like the images in this book and would like to investigate using them
for publishing, promotions or advertising, please visit our website
www.practicalpictures.com for more information.

Publisher: Joanna Lorenz
Editorial Director: Judith Simons
Project Editors: Katy Bevan and Molly Perham
Designer: Whitelight
Photography: John Freeman – assisted by Alex Dow
Make-up: Bettina Graham
Illustrator: Samantha Elmhurst
Production Controller: Claire Rae

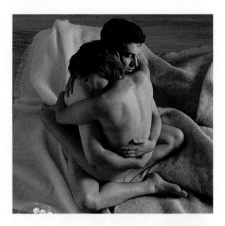

ETHICAL TRADING POLICY
At Anness Publishing we believe that business should be conducted in an ethical and
ecologically sustainable way, with respect for the environment and a proper regard to the
replacement of the natural resources we employ.
As a publisher, we use a lot of wood pulp in high-quality paper for printing, and that wood
commonly comes from spruce trees. We are therefore currently growing more than 750,000
trees in three Scottish forest plantations: Berrymoss (130 hectares/320 acres), West Touxhill
(125 hectares/305 acres) and Deveron Forest (75 hectares/185 acres). The forests we
manage contain more than 3.5 times the number of trees employed each year in making
paper for the books we manufacture.
Because of this ongoing ecological investment programme, you, as our customer, can have
the pleasure and reassurance of knowing that a tree is being cultivated on your behalf to
naturally replace the materials used to make the book you are holding.
Our forestry programme is run in accordance with the UK Woodland Assurance Scheme
(UKWAS) and will be certified by the internationally recognized Forest Stewardship Council
(FSC). The FSC is a non-government organization dedicated to promoting responsible
management of the world's forests. Certification ensures forests are managed in an
environmentally sustainable and socially responsible way. For further information about this
scheme, go to www.annesspublishing.com/trees

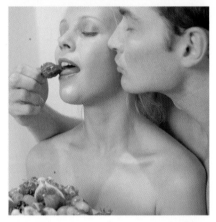

A CIP catalogue record for this book is available from the British Library.

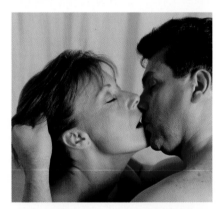

Previously published as *Great Sex for Long-Term Lovers*

PUBLISHER'S NOTE
Although the advice and information in this book are believed to be accurate and true at the
time of going to press, neither the authors nor the publisher can accept any legal
responsibility or liability for any errors or omissions that may have been made nor for any
inaccuracies nor for any loss, harm or injury that comes about from following instructions or
advice in this book.

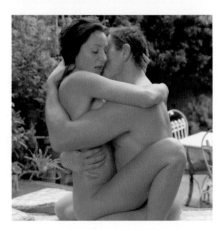

contents

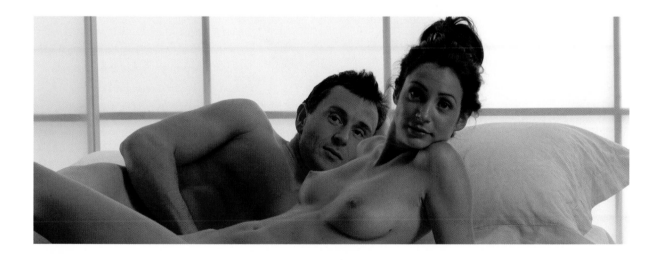

introduction

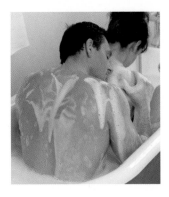

THIS PAGE | Great sex is about exploring your own as well as your partner's sensuality.

WHEN YOU HAVE BEEN with the same partner for some time, sex can become predictable and over-familiar — in fact, modern life is often so stressful and busy that making love tends to take a back seat. The demands of work or family life may be so time-consuming that sex is relegated to a quick cuddle before falling into exhausted sleep. But no matter how long you have been together, it is never too late to change things for the better. This book is aimed at lovers who are in long-term relationships to help them to improve and spice up their sex lives.

Retaining an element of spontaneity is one of the keys to a successful long-term relationship. Just breaking the pattern of ordinary day-to-day life can ratchet up the libido. Taking sex out of the bedroom into the bathroom, the kitchen, or even out of doors will add an element of surprise and

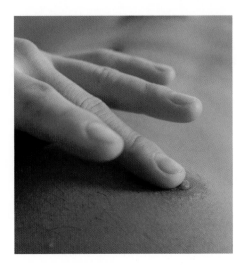

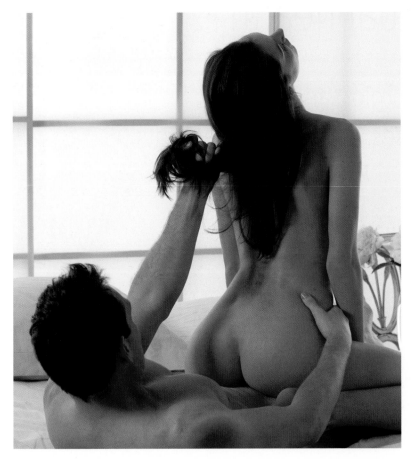

keep your relationship exciting. Appetites for food are similar to those associated with sex, so integrating food into your lovemaking can lead to explosive results.

As you become more spontaneous and adventurous in your lovemaking, you may wish to try advanced techniques to keep your relationship even more exciting. Some of the most famous ancient sex manuals originated in India many hundreds of years ago, but their teachings have a valid place in the sexuality of Western lovers today. The first, the Kama Sutra, has an uninhibited approach to sexual passion that is more enlightening than the theories of many modern-day erotologists. It describes in great detail the delicacy of foreplay and the importance of both partners being satisfied sexually. It was followed by the Ananga Ranga and later by Tantric philosophy, both of which have used the Kama Sutra in their teaching as a sexual blueprint, adapting the positions and practices.

Sex usually gets better as you grow older. Maturity does not mean that you don't need the same physical and emotional intimacy that you demanded when you were young. Intimacy is an important part of your life at any age. In fact, it can help you live longer if you have an active sex life because lovemaking is a workout in itself. Regular exercise promotes energy and stamina. If you are feeling good about yourself and your body, then you can feel good about your sex life, whatever age you happen to be. There are many kinds of exercise you can try — just taking a walk in the open air together whenever you can will keep you in shape. Yoga and Pilates are particularly beneficial forms of exercise for both men and women as they increase suppleness and flexibility, which makes for great sex.

At some point during your life your sexual activity may be inhibited for physical or emotional

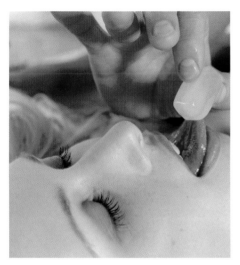

reasons. A temporary loss of libido is very common in long relationships. Men may have ejaculation problems and women may suffer from pain while having sex. Such problems can be devastating for both partners, and it is crucial to keep the lines of communication open by discussing things openly and lovingly between you. If necessary, enlist the help of your doctor or a sex therapist – useful addresses are given at the back of this book.

You need to keep working at your sexual relationship throughout your life, just as you need to keep working at the rest of your relationship. Practice makes perfect. We are all students of sex, and even the greatest lovers have something to learn. Learning does not start and stop with a book. It begins with your partner and is a long exciting journey that you take together, venturing into each other's minds and sensuality. Your travels should take you both into uncharted territory, discovering what makes each other tick, and how to capture the essence of your loved one.

Hopefully, by dipping into this inspiring reference book, and enjoying what you read, you will find something that you and your partner can use together to help make your sex life better and more exciting.

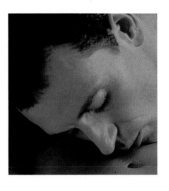

THIS PAGE | Sensuality is about sight, smell, touch, sound and taste.

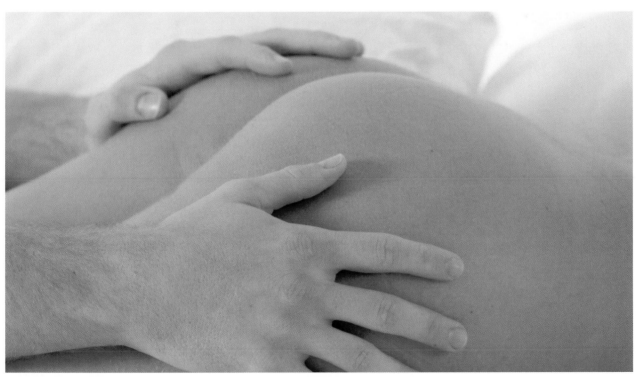

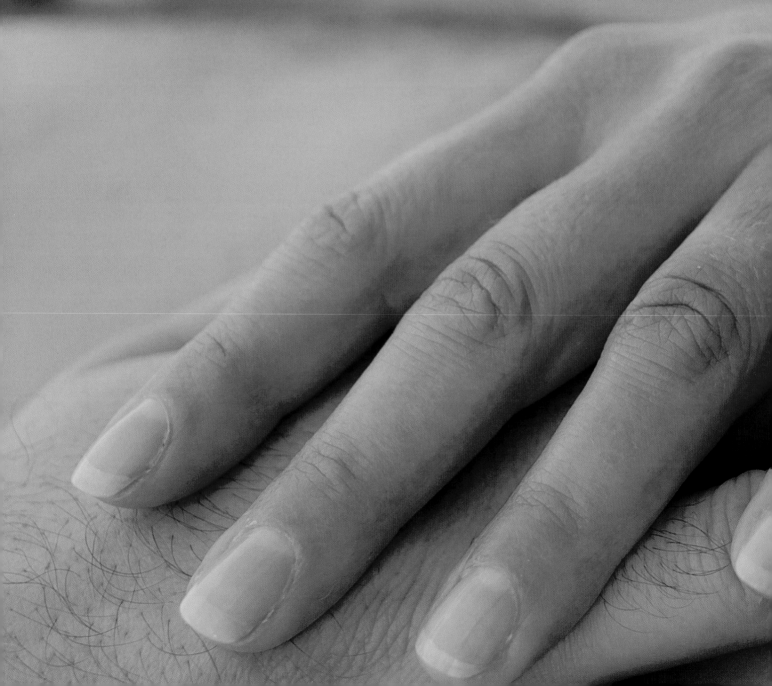

seasons of love

A long-term relationship is constantly subject to change, with ebbs and flows, ups and downs. As you journey through your lives together your relationship changes and matures, as do the seasons of the year, from the exciting, carefree years of early spring to the more laid back and contented golden winter years. Your sexual needs and desires follow these ebbs and flows, but are the essence of what keeps your relationship youthful and timeless.

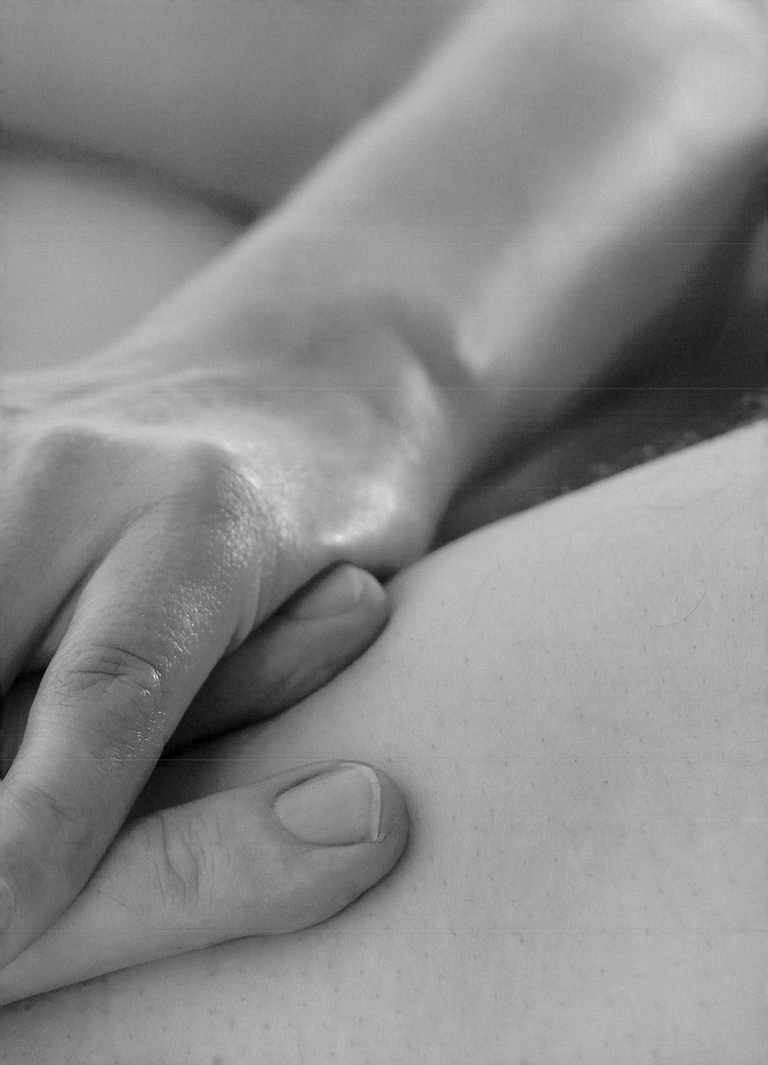

long-term lovers

A RELATIONSHIP CAN BE LIKENED TO THE SEASONS of the year, with spring, summer, autumn and winter each bringing with them their own qualities and climatic changes. Even the strongest relationships tend to be cyclical, with ups and downs, good times and bad. This is worth remembering as you go through your journey together, so that when there are stormy bad times, you can weather them by looking forward to better, sunnier times to come.

spring

The season of spring is the beginning of your relationship with your partner, the first few years when you meet, fall in love, before you decide whether to marry or cohabit. This is often the most carefree time, in which you spend a lot of time getting to know one another and allowing your roots to entwine, building the foundations on which you will grow as a team. With little to tie you, this is often a romantic season in which you feel truly secure in the knowledge that you will cope with anything life throws at you, because you have each other.

Springtime sex lives are exciting and adventurous. You can rarely take your hands off one another and use every spare moment together in making love and being romantic. If things become tougher in the future, it will be this era that you will refer back to. You will be able to

RIGHT AND BELOW | In the springtime of your relationship, you are endlessly fascinated with your lover and want to be with them all the time.

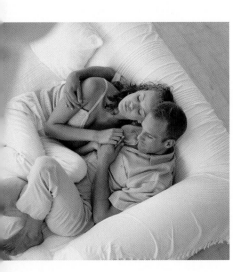

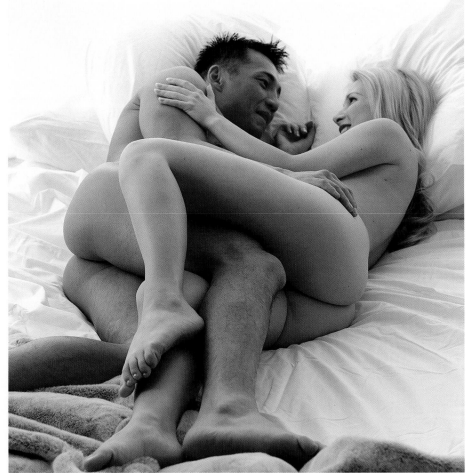

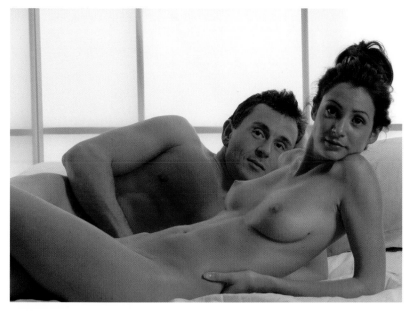
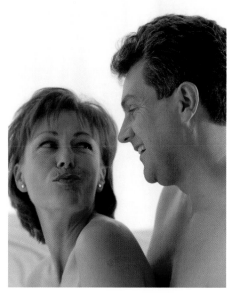

remind each other of how much love you have shared – you are building a scrapbook of memories that you can call on in the future.

summer

The summer of a relationship signifies a settling down period in which you begin to build a nest, find a home together, plan your futures and realize your dreams. Deciding on children will cause you both to re-evaluate your priorities over careers, social lives and sex lives. Sex changes during this season, as the emphasis is upon making love and creating another human being together, rather than having sex just for fun. Having a baby together is one of the most powerful and bonding things any two people can do. With a bit of time both of you will adjust to the changes and enjoy your new roles as mum and dad, providing you don't ignore the fact that you are also still lovers with sexual needs and desires.

autumn

Autumn is represented as the time when the kids fly the nest and lovers return to being just two again. This can be a difficult time for parents who have devoted the last couple of decades to their children. It is difficult to remember what life was like before the children came on the scene, and so it is important that a couple discuss the issues well

in advance. This is a time to plan your future together once again, to start talking about retirement and to make plans to finally fulfil your long-term dreams. Sexually this is a time of rediscovery, confirming each other's sexuality and using the stability and confidence in yourself and each other that you have built over the years to create better sex.

winter

The onset of winter signifies the beginning of another distinct, golden season as you share your retirement and, for many, grandchildren. You can enjoy each other's company with all the stresses and strains of work and dependent children finally put behind you. Most people do not associate senior citizens with sexuality, but in many cases this is an important and precious aspect of a long-standing relationship. You may no longer be swinging from the chandeliers but sex and touch are still important. Although there may be more health challenges to face as you age and libidos may not be what they once were, romance and seduction never age. By continuing to regard each other and your relationship as challenging and fun, you can maintain excitement and indulge each other with the frivolity that the freedom of old age can bring, working together to make your relationship both timeless and ageless.

ABOVE LEFT AND ABOVE | In the summer and autumn of your relationship you can face anything if you keep communicating.

BELOW | The romance doesn't have to fade with the years.

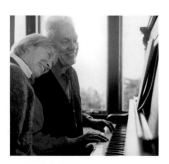

settling down

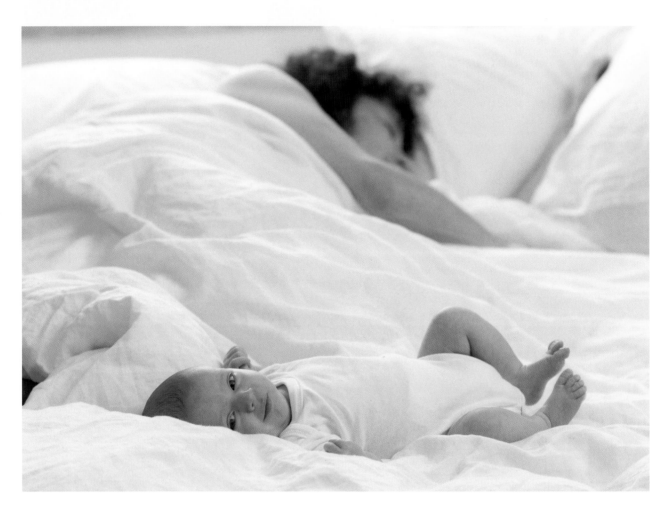

ABOVE | For many couples a long-term relationship is a welcome reprieve from the singles circuit. However, once you decide to start a family, your bed will never be your own again.

FOR MOST COUPLES, the first few years of marriage or cohabitation are an exciting time. You have finally escaped the dating scene and are confident and content that you have discovered the person who makes you happy. This can be a unique time for many relationships where you can concentrate on each other's sexual needs without any other forms of distraction, such as children or responsibility for elderly parents. The next stage for many couples is starting a family. This said, the introduction of a third set of feet in your home brings with it a total rearrangement of your priorities, your social life and, yes, your sex life.

Sex is often the last thing on the minds of new parents, until their baby settles into a routine of sleeping through the night. There are numerous

emotional problems that are common to almost every couple during this time. New mothers can become both physically and emotionally exhausted. Many feel their role as a sexual woman has been totally replaced by that of a child-bearer who is constantly cleaning, feeding, bathing and nurturing her new baby, with no time for nurturing herself. Men may feel neglected or even left out of this new regime. These are all very common issues that new parents face as their lives go through one of the biggest transitions. It's important to remember that these changes are occurring to you as a couple and not as individuals and you need to talk about it together.

During your child's early years they will require a lot of your time and attention and it is all too

sex during pregnancy and after the birth

With a normal, healthy pregnancy, there is absolutely no reason why you should not continue to have a normal, healthy sex life, unless advised otherwise by your doctor. You cannot hurt the baby, who is comfortably cushioned in the amniotic fluid. As the pregnancy progresses, man-on-top positions are likely to become uncomfortable, even impossible. Experiment with positions that suit the two of you. "Spoons" is often a favourite and some women favour rear entry positions. It is a myth that lovemaking will bring on a premature labour, although there is some evidence that substances present in semen may encourage labour at full-term.

For reasons of health, women are usually advised not to have penetrative sex for six weeks after giving birth. If an episiotomy scar hurts or the birth itself was very painful, a woman may be afraid that lovemaking will also hurt. Adapting the Extended Sexual Orgasm technique, combined with gentleness and patience, will probably overcome this. If she is breastfeeding, sore or cracked nipples may mean this is definitely not an erogenous zone. This is a difficult time for men as well, who may be tired after waking with the baby in the night if you are taking turns. This is a major life adjustment for both of you – sharing the burden together will unite you.

easy to put your sex life to one side, or neglect the need for time out to be a couple. Try to set aside some time once a week to make a date with each other. Get a babysitter or ask grandparents to take the kids once a week. Use this time to get out of the house and spend some romantic time together discussing issues that have been on your mind, but try to avoid constantly discussing your children. This is a perfect opportunity to talk freely about sex and how you can both work to improve things. If the kids can stay away overnight from time to time it's even better, as you can enjoy each other in a more uninhibited manner.

families today

There are many different relationships and family structures nowadays that work equally as well as the stereotypical married couple. Many couples prefer to remain unmarried, even though they have a family together, and some couples even choose to live apart as they can be a happier unit when they are together by keeping their own space. More same-sex couples are setting up home together and choosing to adopt children or find surrogate mothers or fathers or sperm donors, to help them have their own.

Relationships can be complicated whichever sexual path you follow. Not all couples who get together stay together for the rest of their lives. Often people separate or divorce and begin a life

with a new person. Starting again with someone new, when either you or your partner already have kids from a past relationship, can be tricky as you have to integrate yourself or your partner into a ready-made family. Children are understandably fiercely loyal to both their parents and so often a new partner on the scene can cause problems.

Children of blended families (couples who both have children) and stepchildren will invariably need plenty of reassurance and understanding when a new relationship begins. Any stresses and strains in a relationship will affect its sex life. Ultimately, given time, much joy and happiness can be found in these kinds of relationships.

One of the most important roles of a parent is to make sure that your children become confident and unafraid of sex and their developing sexuality. This can be harder than it seems and much of their attitude towards it will stem from how you react to their questions.

It is very common for children to walk in while you are making love, and you need to prepare for it before it happens or else you may react in a way that you will regret. Try just covering up slowly, without making it appear like you were doing something that you shouldn't. Often children think that sex looks like "daddy was hurting mummy" and so it is important to emphasize that what you were doing was positive, and something that two people do when they love each other.

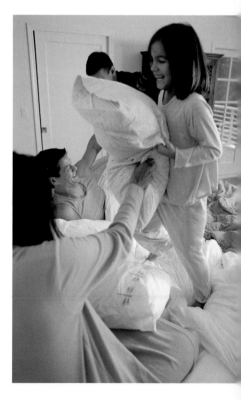

ABOVE | Family life can often be a battle – but making time for a healthy sex life will help maintain the balance in the equation.

empty nesters

IF YOU HAVE CHILDREN, then sometime you will experience the "Empty Nest Syndrome". One or all of your babies will have flown away – to university, jobs or into marriage – and you are left alone in your house with your partner. This period in your life often creeps up on you and you don't realize the impact until it happens. What was a longed-for dream of more time together may turn out to be a period of incredible emotional emptiness until you get used to the absence of the children and to spending so much time together.

Once you get used to the idea, it can be a very exciting time. If your sex life has been on the back burner for some years, now is the time to get to know each other again and become sexually reacquainted. You have more time and tend to be more relaxed and positive about having sex.

Another aspect of having more leisure time is that there will be more time to exercise. Whilst physically you will be slowing down, this is a great opportunity to take control and become fitter – start going to those yoga classes! This is crucial because as we age, we need to remain active, not only for our health but also for a good sex life.

time of life
It is the period when women may be going through the menopause, the end of their reproductive life. This causes emotional and physical challenges, so talk to your partner about how it makes you feel so he understands the process. Many women find that taking HRT (hormone replacement therapy) can help them through this period of change – lessening the hot

RIGHT AND OPPOSITE | Once the kids have flown the nest, you will have more time to spend alone with each other.

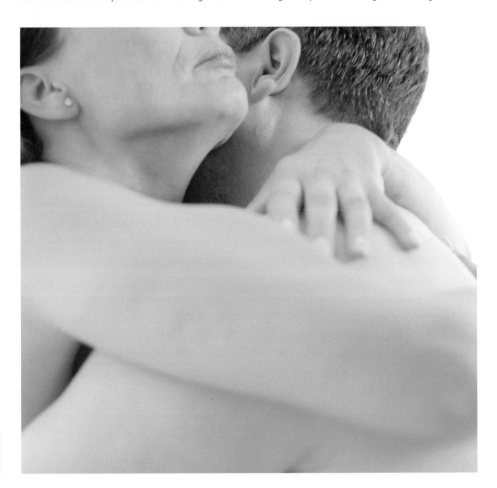

flushes, mood swings and forgetfulness. Sexual desire or libido varies greatly in every woman whether pre- or post-menopausal. Hormone levels determine sex drive and diminished hormone levels undoubtedly interfere with sexual desire. Although oestrogen plays a part, the hormone that has been shown to be most closely associated with sex drive is testosterone. The ovary, although capable of producing oestrogen after a "natural" menopause, may continue to produce significant amounts of testosterone for several years. This is the reason why many women maintain a good sex drive for a considerable length of time. These testosterone levels provide additional benefits to the naturally menopausal woman. Tissues of the body are able to convert some of this circulating testosterone to oestrogen.

When women undergo a hysterectomy where the ovaries are also removed, this benefit may be lost. Some women even find that their sexual desire increases after menopause (if their ovaries are left) as they are free from pain and excessive bleeding.

mid-life crisis

Men also may well be experiencing a slow-down in their sexual response time, taking longer to become aroused as they approach middle age. In fact, both men and women may need more stimulation to become aroused and to orgasm. But, since you will hopefully be able to spend more time together, take advantage of this. Talk to each other about what pleases you. If you have difficulty communicating, or are not able to take that step forward together, then you may well need to speak to a therapist.

It is at this stage that men may have a "mid-life crisis". This can manifest itself in seeking reinforcement in a younger girlfriend or a new motorbike when he normally drives a family car. This is just a glance back at his youth and women often have similar feelings. Patience is required during this time, on the part of both of you. It can be frightening to let go of the younger part of you that you are accustomed to – however, you are exchanging it for the confidence and experience that can only come with age.

looking lively

It is important for both men and women to make an effort to look attractive for their partner and for their own self-respect. Perhaps you can get into the routine of spending an hour or so having a long bath and pampering yourself. Invest in some glamorous nightwear that makes you feel sensuous. Give yourselves the time to feel sexy as adults and not just parents or workers.

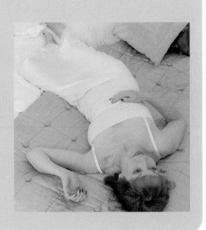

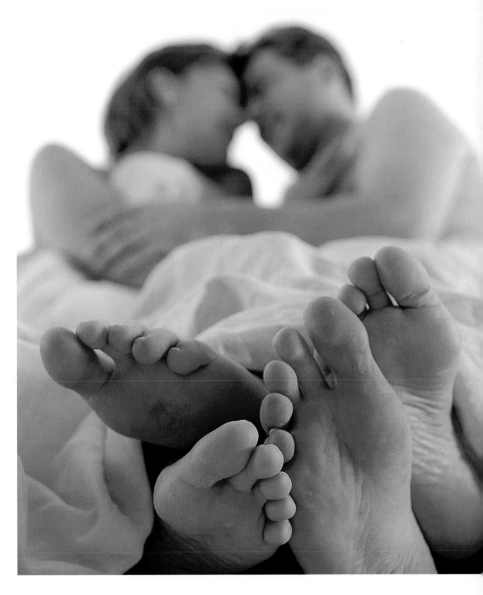

golden years

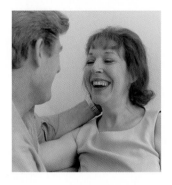

IT IS A MYTH THAT YOU STOP HAVING SEX when you are in your "golden years". Just because you are older, it does not mean that you don't need the same physical and emotional intimacy that you demanded when you were young. Intimacy is an important part of your life at any age.

An active sex life will keep you mentally fit and healthy, and having a good companion whom you can share your life with is said to be the key to living longer. The emphasis on the necessity of regular exercise promoted over the last couple of decades means that older people will be fitter than ever. Having a positive attitude is crucial for a good sex life. Your body may be aging, but for many, your desires certainly aren't. If you are experiencing problems having erections on a long-term basis, you can ask your doctor for their advice. Older men may need some more stimulation in order to achieve erection – a little manual assistance is sometimes necessary. In these cases oral sex and mutual masturbation can be an enjoyable path to explore together. The time that you make love can be an important factor in later years as well. It is frequently recommended

ABOVE AND BELOW | Companionship has many mutual benefits.

RIGHT | Taking up a hobby, like dancing, with your partner can be one way to rekindle romance.

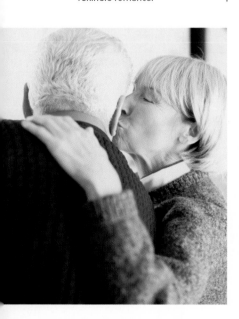

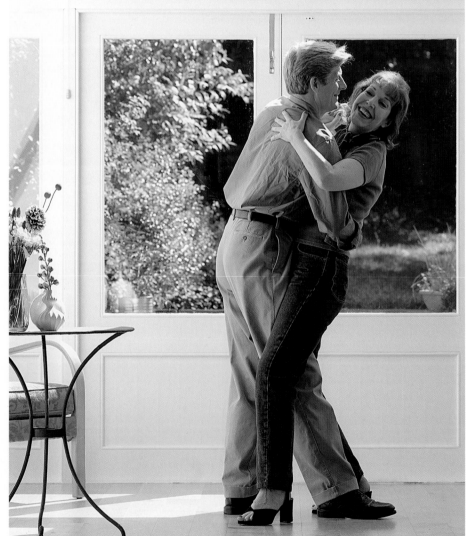

that older adults should try making love in the morning, as older men are more likely to have a firm erection in the morning after a good night's sleep. There are also unexpected advantages for men as you get older; you can delay ejaculation for longer, and your partner will love you for this.

freedom years

By their golden years, women have finished with the menopause and can experience a new sense of sexual liberation. There are some physiological changes of course such as vaginal lubrication, which instead of taking only 15 to 30 seconds when younger can now take up to five minutes. There are plenty of lubricants, and even hormonal treatments that can help. Women who continue to have sex after the menopause finishes will remain fitter and their vaginas will remain more elastic than those women who do not.

A woman's sex drive over the age of 65 is more stable than a man's. In fact a woman reaches her peak in her late twenties or thirties and remains on that plateau until her sixties. A woman of 80 has the same physical potential for orgasm as a woman of 20.

Even if sexual desire has abated, intimacy is still an important part of any loving relationship, regardless of age. Touching and cuddling up together and learning how to massage each other can be extremely sensual. Setting aside time to visit galleries together or to go for long walks – perhaps joining a dance class – can give you that extra contact outside the home that you need. To stay young you have to feel young, regardless of what your body is doing. Being active together, and remaining tactile with each other, will help to keep your relationship as fresh and exciting as in the early days when you had only just met each other.

going it alone

As women tend to live longer than men, the major problem is often having a partner to share their sexuality with. Many older people have to come to terms with the loss of their loved one and one of the important issues is how you deal with the loss of intimacy and sex that was part of a

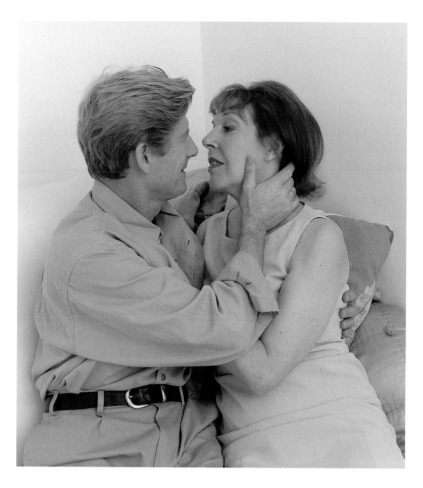

loving relationship. Sexual desire and drive do not die with your partner. Masturbation can be especially helpful in these circumstances and will help you to keep your sexual identity and sexuality alive.

You are never too old to fall in love, and on a happier note, many older people can find new love and companionship in their golden years. This can bring comfort to them, their new partners and their extended families alike.

Society's image of "old people" is that they are too sagging, wrinkly and unattractive to even think about having a sex life. It is up to all of us to resist subscribing to that kind of agism, not just mature people themselves, but also younger generations. As the baby-boomer generation comes of age, attitudes will surely have to change – there are going to be a lot of healthy pensioners out there.

We owe it to our children and those who come after us to claim our sexuality in old age. If we don't do it, how will they?

ABOVE | Mature couples have more time to themselves to rekindle the eroticism of their early relationship.

rediscovery

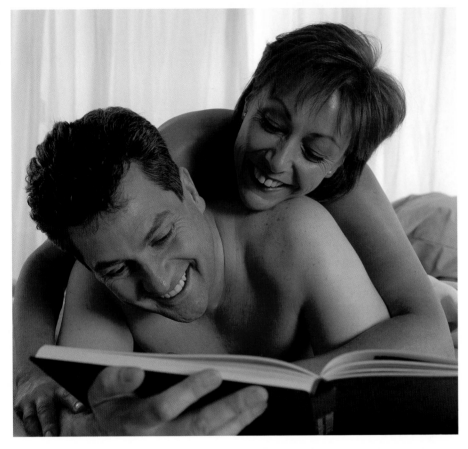

ABOVE | Life is tough and sometimes your sex life can suffer, becoming dull or non-existent. It is time to take action, read a book about sex together and share your laughter.

THERE INEVITABLY COMES A TIME in most couples' lives when the emphasis of their relationship is no longer on sex, and in fact has not been for quite some time. It is easy for this to happen to couples who have been together for a while and have devoted their partnership to their kids, careers, home-building and the multitude of other tasks, whatever their age. Standard patterns and routines somehow appear over the years, often without you realizing it. Sex may be dull, and many feel that they have worn out the possibility of having exciting, exhilarating sensual sex again.

It is never too late to reawaken each other's sensuality. Good sex is the magic ingredient to a great relationship. There is joy in store for some, perhaps discovering orgasm for the first time after a lifetime of frustration and disappointment. To get all your sexual fantasies fulfilled in the later stages of a relationship can be heartening. The lesson is that it is never too late to start.

Rediscovering your own and your partner's sexuality is a journey through known territory that will invariably lead you to a new destination. Remember a particular place where you both felt passionate – revisit it. If there is a particular song that invokes special memories for you both, play it while you cuddle or massage each other. Perhaps there is one dish or type of wine that reminds you of a particularly memorable evening. Each of these may reawaken the spontaneity that you may have lost over the years, but the main focus should be on setting aside some time for you both to talk and appreciate each other's needs and wants.

The biggest erogenous zone is the brain, so this is a good place to start stimulating each other's sensuality. Talk to each other, avoiding selfless topics such as the children. Visit museums or cinemas together, share interesting extracts from a book, or create meals together in a new style.

practical steps

The following are some hints and tips that couples can incorporate into their relationship to help them to rediscover each other's sexuality, and their own. An understanding of trust and respect is paramount in all loving relationships, and as you age and mature together you need to develop an element of flexibility to allow for personal growth and development. This may involve taking practical steps to nurture, listen and act on one another's needs:

● Talk to your partner about making time for lovemaking and if you lead very busy lives, clear a space in the diary. Don't rush sexual activity and make time for the post-coital cuddles, too.

● You may well both be feeling horny at different times, so that will have to be negotiated. There's no prescribed perfect frequency of lovemaking – how often you do it, or how infrequently – it just has to work for both of you.

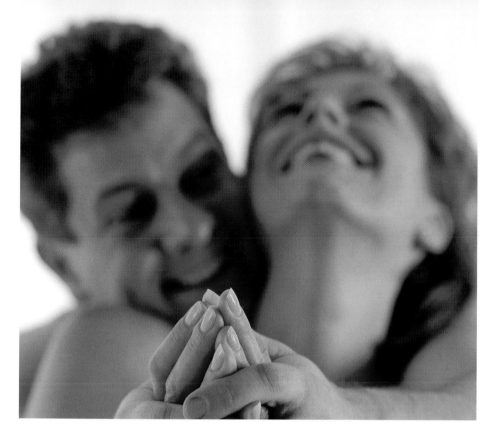

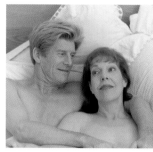

ABOVE | No matter how long you have been together, it is never too late to change things for the better.

LEFT | Trying something new together might end up just being a laugh, but then wasn't that part of the idea?

● Talk about sexual fantasies together and see whether it is possible to carry some of them out. If you find you are falling into a routine, take stock and try something different for a change. "How about trying this today?"

● Many people see sex as a way of making up after an argument, which can be very exciting, as well as an easy way of keeping emotionally close to their partner. But the potential for misunderstanding the real problem that caused the argument in the first place is enormous. Try to understand how you both function emotionally, talk about it and see how you can progress.

● Many people feel that they are not fully satisfying their lover and worry about it. Make yourself feel better by addressing some of the things that concern you and discuss your sexual performance with your partner, asking them how you can make sex better for them.

● Familiarity can breed contempt in a long-term relationship, so try to retain some of the mystery and your own personal privacy. For example, the bathroom can be a great place to shower and bath together but it should also be a private space sometimes. You need to be able to tell each other when you need some privacy and your own separate space and time.

● And lastly, be romantic and thoughtful towards each other. Kiss each other before you say goodbye and when you see each other again. Remember the thank yous and the small pleasantries. Buy each other small gifts or tokens – after all, it's the little things that matter.

keeping the bedroom hot

Here's how to maintain the spice:

● Use soft sexy music, dim lighting and candles or try covering the bed and floor with rose petals to create a more sensual space.

● Reorganize the bedroom every now and again to make a change in the surroundings – perhaps move the bed to a different position or bring in furniture from other rooms.

● Brighten up the room with flowers, or change some of the pictures in the photo frames. You could even buy a new print or painting to hang on the walls.

● Use sexy bed linen, perhaps silk sheets or a new bed-throw of fake fur.

● Experiment using different coloured light bulbs or change your net curtains for lightly-dyed sheer fabric: a change of light intensity or colour can completely alter the ambience of a room.

● If you have a television in the room, try taking it out for a while. A recent study showed that couples were having more sex in the 1950s than they are today, and one of the reasons was because of today's reliance on television for entertainment. By taking it out of the bedroom you will have to be creative and work on entertaining each other in different ways.

long-term tactics

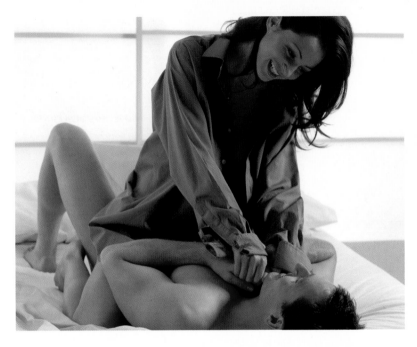

ABOVE | Your relationship with your loved one should be fun.

sex appeal

Rediscovering your sex appeal is about building your confidence. If you feel ashamed or embarrassed about your body then you will not be able to go full throttle during sex. If your body image is inhibiting your sex life then you have to take positive steps to do something about it.

Start doing more exercise; take time to dress up, wear sexy underwear. Go out together somewhere smart that requires you both to dress up a bit.

SOME OF THE MOST SUCCESSFUL long-term relationships cite humour and being best friends as the essential ingredients that make it work. Great friendship involves respectful behaviour towards each other, friendly gestures, lots of touching and cuddling and of course good sex. If you can have a great laugh together as well, all the better. A loving relationship should be a mutual appreciation society, to coin a phrase. Respect your differences and remember, you can't change the other person. Only they can change themselves.

Studies show that laughter is seriously good for your health. It lowers blood pressure, reduces stress and boosts your immune system. It also triggers the release of endorphins, chemicals that provide a natural painkiller for the body, and produce that "feel-good factor".

If we all looked at the physical mechanics of the way people make love, the mess they get themselves into, the funny faces they pull when having an orgasm, the fumbling, farting and funny noises that emanate from the bed, no one would ever be able to keep a straight face while having sex. Although sex is seriously fun, it has its

ridiculous side. There's a good reason why we say that laughter is the best medicine and this applies equally to your sexual relationship.

buying gifts

Buying each other sexy gifts is another fantastic way of reawakening each other's sexuality. Everyone loves both receiving and giving gifts, especially if they are spontaneous. Men can buy their partner some sexy lingerie or underwear from specialist boutiques. It is important that he buys something that will suit her taste – if in doubt then ask the shop assistant, they are usually only too keen to help! It is important also to buy it in the right context. If he buys it because he secretly wants her to look more sexy, or feels that their sex life is boring and wants to spice it up, she will invariably pick up on this and may feel offended or hurt. A better approach is for him to gently discuss with her beforehand the possibility of spicing things up, saying things like: "I would really love to spend more time with you sexually, perhaps we can try some new things together." Then she will be more prepared for her new gift, and the likelihood is that it will be better received.

More adventurous gifts such as dildos, vibrators and other sex toys must also be handled with sensitivity. If a couple has got into a pattern of rather repetitive and mundane sex and then one springs a vibrator on the other, it may be a bit of a shock, regardless of the intentions. Again, it is important to establish through discussion that you both want to try something new – there's no room here for unilateral action.

sex talk

For some reason couples often find talking about sex together really difficult regardless of how long they have been together. One reason for this may be that although sex is something that you do together, often the experience is pretty personal. During orgasm, for example, individuals often disappear temporarily into their own intense world of pleasure, and even building up to orgasm requires an element of personal concentration.

Another reason couples may find it tricky to talk about sex is fear that they may upset or offend their partner by telling them what they like, and, more importantly, what they do not like. This is especially true for couples in long-term relationships who may have spent years doing it in a specific way that is not necessarily giving one or both of them enough satisfaction.

The important thing to remember is that when you love one another, the need to satisfy and please each other sexually is crucial. All you need to do is approach the subject sensitively, avoiding direct criticism. A good technique is to use the question and answer method. When you are in bed together, spend time trying to rediscover areas of sensuality on your partner's body by asking questions such as "May I touch you here?" or "Can I stroke you there?" The recipient should avoid responding with negative responses such as "No that feels awful." Try "That feels great, but if you do it this way it feels even better."

A tricky situation is when your partner is doing something to you that you really don't like, but are unsure how to deal with it without hurting them. Try focusing on the positive by saying things such as "I like it when you do that but I much prefer it when you do this", or "I love giving you a blow-job and I love the way you taste, but I find it uncomfortable when you thrust too deeply into my mouth, perhaps we could try a different position."

BELOW LEFT | Don't force anything on your partner you feel they won't like.

BELOW | Make a pact to buy each other something you would like them to try: "I have heard that using a vibrator during sex can be really fun, I'm quite keen to try this, what do you think about it?" Even if they are not keen, the door has been opened for a discussion on their sex life.

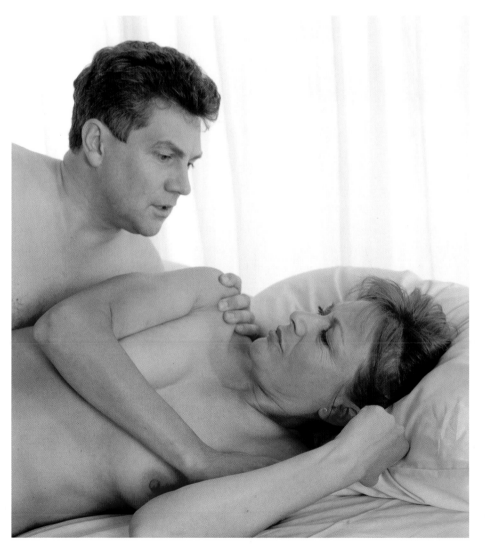

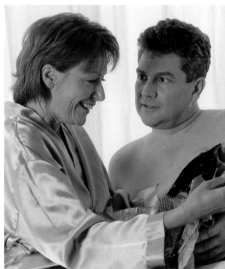

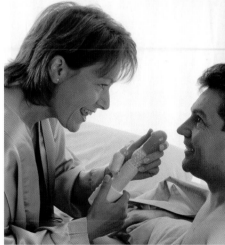

talking and listening

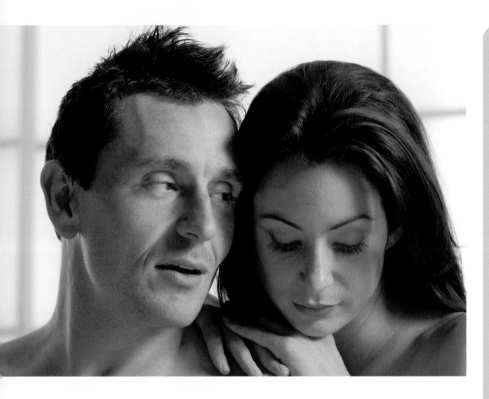

ABOVE | Making a connection with your partner is more than just a physical thing – talking and listening are crucial to keep a relationship strong and healthy. If you stop communicating, things can only get worse.

ONE OF THE MAIN PROBLEMS that couples experiencing difficulty have in common is an inability to talk effectively. Communication is the key to getting what you want out of a relationship. If done with sufficient sensitivity, it can help you to air grievances with one another and to stop one partner doing something that the other feels is annoying, hurtful or aggravating. Communication is a learned skill and blocks often occur from situations that have happened in an individual's past. It is important that each couple works together to find out what their communication strengths and weaknesses are in order to understand what makes them react to each other in the way that they do.

learning to listen

Listening is paramount in successful communication. Often people who do not listen to their partners find themselves cutting in on them, or remaining silent. Inwardly they may be thinking about what they are going to say next, without actually paying attention to what their partner is saying. Listening is one of the most valuable skills that a therapist can teach. Often couples learn this by noting how their therapist listens to each of them when they speak, and the positive effect this has on them. Therapists can encourage individuals to listen more openly and not to feel defensive when their partner is speaking, thus reducing the need to attack. By listening, couples learn to give each other time for self-expression, taking away the bad feeling or resentment that is engendered when we believe we are not being heard.

Some of the listening techniques that counsellors may advise are as follows:
● Give your full attention to your partner when they are talking by focusing on their face and voice.
● If other thoughts intrude into your mind allow them to gradually fade as you gently swing your attention back round to what is being said to you.

• Once they have finished, don't jump in immediately, give yourself a couple of seconds to evaluate what has been said and ultimately make them feel like you are taking stock of what they have been saying to you.

• Listening is not all about being quiet and maintaining eye contact, it is also about encouraging your partner to speak and open up to you. The person listening should try to keep their body language as open as possible by turning towards their partner and not blocking them with gestures. They should keep their face turned towards them and look interested in what they are saying.

• Acknowledgement signals are very helpful, a nod or encouraging "yes" or "okay" all tell the partner that their words have been heard, and although you may not necessarily agree, you are accepting what they are saying. If they pause, use words that will encourage them to elaborate. Phrases such as "That incident must have made you very angry," or "You must have felt very upset when that happened to you," will help your partner to say more about their feelings and emotions.

talking to each other

Talking is also an important skill that therapists will help couples to learn. When a relationship is in its early stages, couples tend to talk a lot together to learn more about one another. As they continue, this talk becomes less and less since they already know each other and so don't feel the need to ask as much. Conversations can become short-lived and stagnant, discussing mundane issues such as "What do you want for breakfast?" as opposed to "How do you feel this morning?"

The worst thing a couple can do when they talk together is attack one another. Often when people feel passionate about something their choice of words is instantly on the offensive and confrontational, making them feel like they are getting their point across but leaving their partner feeling defensive.

The following are some common phrases and constructions that often trigger arguments, and some alternative ways of addressing the issue that may be less explosive.

blame "You ruined my evening when you told everyone that story." Instead of blaming your partner try to describe how you feel: "I felt uncomfortable and didn't enjoy myself this evening."

accusation "You made me feel furious when you forgot to pay the gas bill." Admit to your feelings by saying: "I feel..." instead of "you made me feel..."

nagging "I have asked you hundreds of times to do the dishes." Try a more constructive approach such as "Shall we do the dishes together?"

shouting Try not to raise your voice and point your finger to get your message across. Shouting will evoke an immediate defensive response. Instead, try using a softer tone and less harsh hand gestures.

a useful exercise

One exercise that can help in understanding blocks to communication is to sit down together with a pad and pen and finish the following sentences:

• A time when I said something that really made a difference was...

• A time when I was afraid or nervous to speak my mind was...

• A time I said something that I later regretted was...

• A time I took the time to listen to someone and really helped them was...

BELOW | Sometimes we need to go back to school, and unlearn some bad habits.

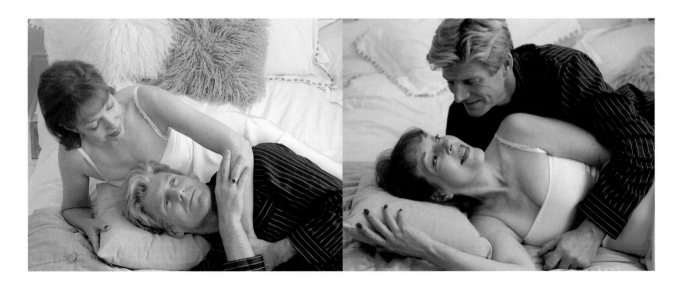

seeking help

COMMUNICATING WITH ONE ANOTHER is one of the most useful tools for ensuring success in a relationship. Sadly, successful communication is not as easy as many people may think. As a relationship progresses and other factors and influences take over such as work pressures and children, many couples find themselves communicating less and less often, unwittingly building barriers that eventually seem impossible to break down.

Therapy and counselling can be a huge benefit here. Many therapists say that a lot of couples come to them thinking that their relationship has already ended and that they have lost faith in their love and are trying therapy as a "last resort". The encouraging news is that all too often this is not the case. The use of sexual and relationship therapy has become increasingly popular as couples are less inclined to settle for an unsatisfactory love life and quite rightly seek to better their alliance on both an emotional and physical level.

The therapist will take time with the couple to re-evaluate the communication skills, find the root of the problem and help them to change their approach to each other so that their conversations become more positive and encouraging. Often communication problems stem from learned patterns picked up as children. A child whose parent was non-communicative or even abusive can carry the emotional effects of this over into their relationship in adult life, often without realizing it. This is a very common problem and once it has been identified, it can be worked through and with the help of the therapist, the couple can begin working on developing more effective methods of communication.

visiting a therapist

The majority of couples who visit a therapist do so because they believe that their relationship is in trouble. Often they are unsure of how bad things

BELOW AND RIGHT | Whatever you do or don't do in bed with your partner, it is crucial to keep the channels of communication open. Masters and Johnson, through their research, popularized the concept of sexual therapy and openly talking about sex.

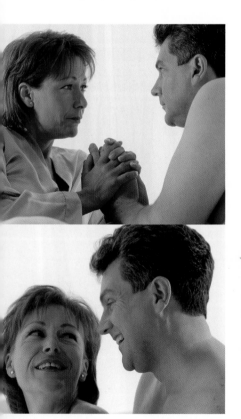

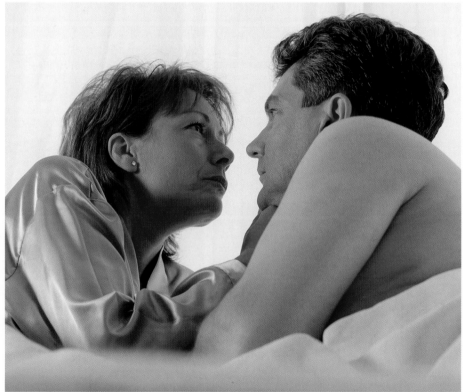

hot off the press

In 1948 Alfred Kinsey published his mass study on the human sexual male, followed in 1953 by that of the female. He shocked America by producing statistics such as 50 per cent of males had cheated on their wives, and 25 per cent of women had done the same to their husbands. *Playboy* hit the news-stands in 1953, and in the 1960s William Masters and Virginia Johnson published the first serious study on the physiology of orgasms and arousal.

In 1976, Shere Hite published *The Hite Report: A Nation-wide Study of Female Sexuality*. Hite's book contained statistical analysis, which was questioned and supported by statisticians and other scientific reviewers alike, causing much academic debate and controversy. It also contained anecdotes from women on their opinions and complaints relating to their sex lives. It became an instant bestseller.

Dr Alex Comfort broke down many barriers in the West with his 1972 publication *The Joy of Sex: a Gourmet Guide to Love Making*. This book and his other later sex manuals allowed couples to explore their sexuality with more freedom and to push out the boundaries without feeling guilty. Studies of sex have come a long way and there is today a constant stream of new information and books, like this one.

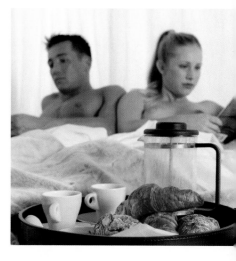

ABOVE | When you wake up with the same person every day, it is hard to maintain any mystery.

BELOW | Try to talk clearly using unthreatening gestures and positive language so you won't start an argument, and remember to listen as well.

are and need an external voice to help them to get back on track. People who no longer feel good about each other or rarely talk except to row have often built up barriers over time that they alone cannot break down.

Relationship support organizations have trained counsellors who will help couples to feel more positive about each other. Choosing and deciding to see a counsellor is often the first and hardest step for any couple experiencing difficulty, and it relies on a real desire from both parties to work together to sort out their problems. Often people are nervous, as they are unsure of what to expect from their first visit. The main purpose of the counsellor will be to provide a safe and supportive environment in which to help you rebuild your relationship. They aim to help you find the external point of reference that you need to see in order to re-evaluate your relationship.

The appointment with the therapist usually takes place in a private room where the couple can relax with the therapist and be guided to talk about their problems. A wide range of approaches and individual techniques are used, so that there is no fixed formula. They look at each individual's past to help provide meanings and answers for problems that may be occurring. They use their interactions and conversations with couples to help highlight or reflect on the roots of some of the problems and they also suggest some practical exercises that couples can try together to take a more active approach towards improving their relationship.

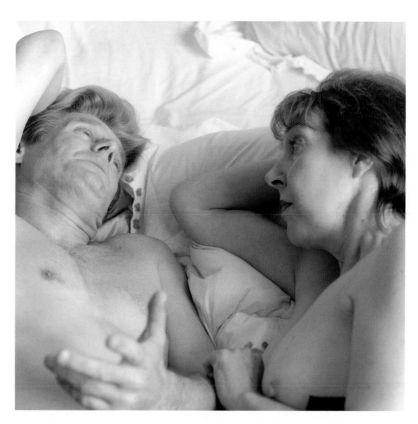

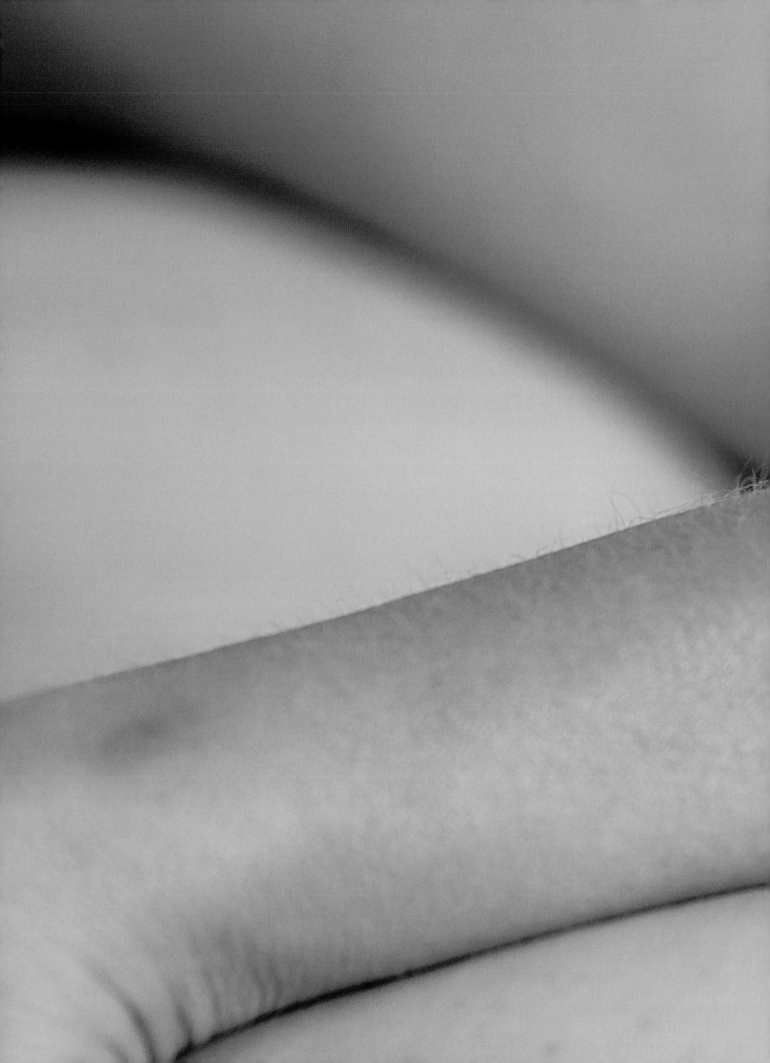

shaking it up

Many long-term relationships experience occasional periods of over-familiarity and predictability. Add some spice and fire to your relationship with some fun and exciting new ideas, allowing you to rediscover both your own and your partner's desire.

out of the bedroom

WHEN YOU HAVE BEEN TOGETHER for a long time, it can be difficult to keep the flames of passion burning brightly, especially if – whether out of habit or because you have children – the only place you have sex is your bedroom. As well as location, give a thought to timing and recall those days when you first met and couldn't keep your hands off each other. If you think about it, making

love after a demanding day at work, cooking dinner and clearing up afterwards, then helping the kids with their homework, will almost certainly be less exciting and, frankly, more of a duty for both of you than rampant sex in the garden shed in the middle of an afternoon's weeding.

One of the most popular alternatives to the bedroom is the bathroom. As there is usually a lock on the door, even if the kids are at home, you are assured of some privacy. Sex in the shower or the bath is extremely sensual, as the hot water stimulates all your touch receptors, making your skin more sensitive. It is also very refreshing and revitalizing. Don't just go for the main event – relish the eroticism of lovingly soaping and rinsing every part of each other's bodies. Concentrating on giving your partner an invigorating body brush will not only produce its own rewards, but will also remind you why your lover's body is so special.

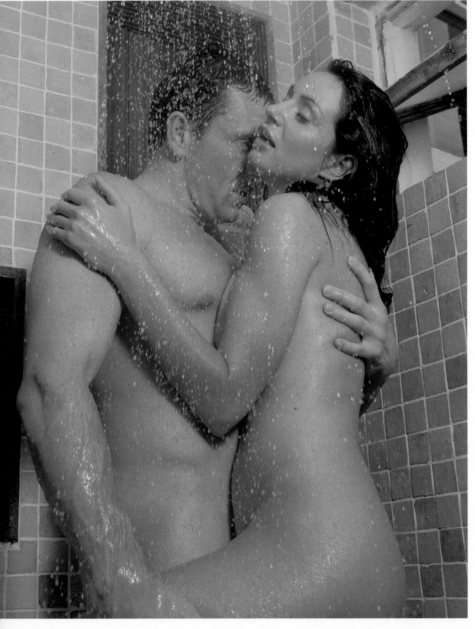

alternative venues

Chairs and sofas are also great places for making love and performing oral sex. Try sitting in your favourite chair in the front room with the curtains and windows open to add an extra notch of excitement and danger. Rocking chairs and recliners are fantastic, as the gentle motion gives a little extra movement to allow deeper penetration.

Cellars and attics are fun because of their secret atmosphere, although a little forethought about cushions and blankets might be a good idea. These places can become your own erotic dens and, if role-play is your thing, then there are unlimited scenarios, from dominatrix dungeons to caveman dwellings.

Stairs are fantastic settings for sex because the different levels allow you to experiment with positions that may otherwise not be possible. The vertical 69 is a challenge to the fittest. The woman sits on the second or third step while her partner kneels on a higher step, so her head is between his legs. Then – very carefully – he manoeuvres his

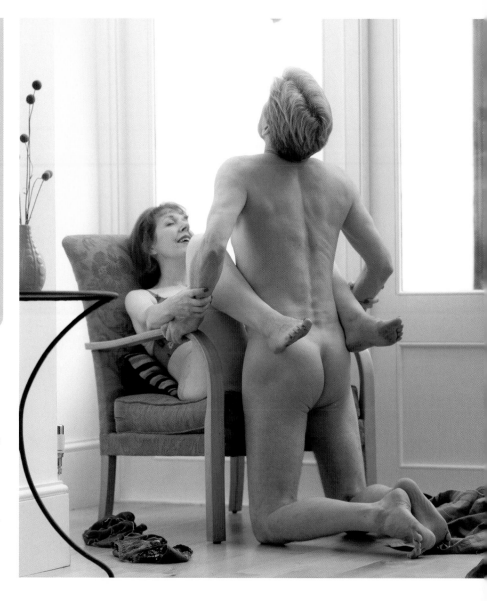

body so that he is head first down the stairs, supporting his weight with his hands on the floor at the bottom of the staircase, with his knees a few steps higher. Underneath him, the woman may need to move slightly or change the step she is on. Both partners' mouths are in contact with the other's genitals.

An easier position is for the man to kneel on the stairs, with the woman sitting one step above, facing him. She can then sit back and hold on to the banisters, while he grasps her by the hips. For additional spice, he can handcuff or tie her wrists to the banisters with a silk scarf and torment her with his hands, tongue and penis.

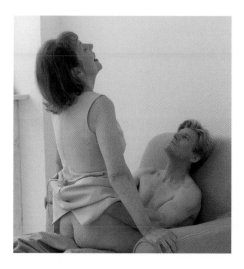

The kitchen, too, offers tasty possibilities. If the woman lies flat on the table and the man stands beside it, supporting her legs straight up in the air, the angle of penetration is intense. If she keeps her legs together, the tightness of her vagina will be immensely exciting for both partners. And, since you are already there, you can explore the possibilities of sensual and sexy foods – whether as an hors d'oeuvre or as a dessert.

There are couples who reckon that making love leaning against or with the woman sitting on an operating washing machine is one of life's truly erotic experiences. The vibration, especially if you time your "cycle" to the final spin, is said to be out of this world.

ABOVE AND LEFT | Chairs and sofas offer comfort as well as scope for some interesting and exciting positions. "Putting your feet up for half an hour" will never have the same meaning again.

the quickie

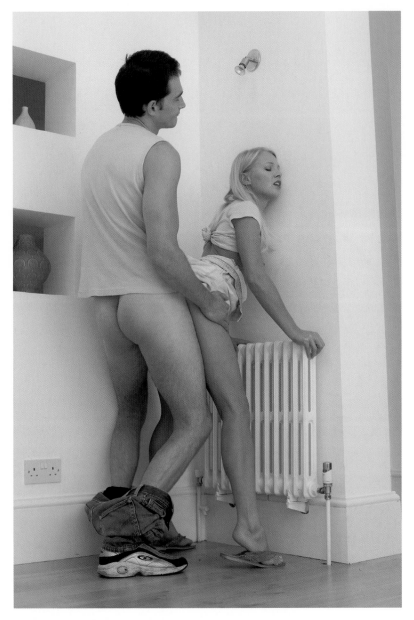

Quickie sex is a wonderfully erotic and lustful way of adding diversity to your love life. Although it cannot and should not replace the long sensual hours of foreplay and lovemaking that are essential in all loving and respectful relationships, it has a place, reaffirming each other's sexuality and reassuring your partner that you still find them the sexiest and most desirable person on the planet. Variety is not described as the spice of life without good reason.

mother of invention

Quick sex is often creative and inventive, two essential ingredients in lovemaking. Creeping up behind your partner while he or she clears the dishes in the kitchen in response to a completely overwhelming lustful urge is both delightful and flattering. There are no limits to when you can do it, whether sneaking off early from a party or a frantic session before you leave for work. It's up to you and your infectious desire.

The bedroom is usually the place where your loving, united encounters take place, so having a quick romp there may undermine the emotional importance of this room. The bathroom, on the other hand, is ideal. Steal in when your partner is having a shower and wordlessly show your intentions by kissing passionately under the hot jets.

ABOVE | Sometimes, the less glamorous the venue, the more exciting the sex.

RIGHT | Surprising your partner in the bathroom can have, well, surprising results.

RETAINING YOUR SENSE OF SPONTANEITY is one of the keys to a successful long-term relationship. It is all too easy to slip into a habitual pattern without noticing, especially when you have family responsibilities, a demanding job and a busy life. Seizing the moment and surprising each other with unplanned flurries of passion keeps excitement and desire alive, adding spice and maintaining the longevity of the relationship.

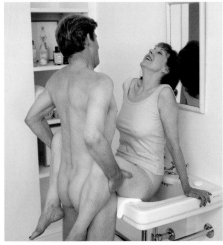

Sometimes the best places are those that seem to be totally unsexy and mundane, such as against a radiator in the front hall. It's almost guaranteed that you will both smile each time you pass that particular radiator in the future. Shamelessly grabbing your partner as soon as they walk through the front door for a passionate encounter on the hall floor is an unmistakable demonstration of your feelings – and who cares if dinner is half an hour late?

The living room is also a great place to have quick, spontaneous sex. While your partner is watching television, why not surprise her with a sexy striptease to distract her? Suddenly blast some music from the stereo as you rip your clothes off in front of her in time to the beat. It's bound to have her in stitches, and laughter is a wonderful aphrodisiac. Alternatively, while he is relaxing in his favourite chair, why not silently hitch up your skirt and sit on his lap, either facing him or facing away, gently moving and rotating your hips until he becomes aroused? It certainly beats making coffee during the advertisement breaks.

timing

If quickie sex is what you have in mind, you do need to choose your moment wisely or the whole idea could backfire. You must also be open and sensitive to your partner's response. Selecting the final five minutes of a nail-biting match on television to give him a blow-job or suggesting steamy bathroom sex when she is in the middle of shaving her legs would be inappropriate. Your partner will either end up "submitting" and feeling exploited and irritable or else push you away and you will feel rejected, unloved and unimportant. Neither of these is conducive to promoting harmony and closeness in your relationship. Quickie sex is, after all, just as much about mutual pleasure as is prolonged, sensual lovemaking – just different. Although being ambushed for a quickie is a great turn-on, sometimes your partner may simply not feel like it and, if they are still unwilling after a little gentle persuasion and encouragement, then it's probably best to postpone the idea until another, rather more suitable moment.

the sky's the limit

Quickie sex does add an element of surprise and keeps your relationship exciting, fun and light-hearted. Just breaking the pattern of day-to-day life can ratchet up the libido for days afterwards.

Nor does quickie sex have to be restricted to the home. If you're feeling reckless – and you really are going to be quick – what about the back seat of the car in a carwash? Try stopping a hotel freight elevator between floors – but watch out for surveillance cameras, there may be penalties for being found out. Airline security permitting, you could go for membership of the Mile High Club. The balcony of a holiday hotel can offer the frisson of exhibitionism without any of the danger, if only the top half of you can be seen. The list is as endless as your imagination – just make sure that you don't get caught *in flagrante*.

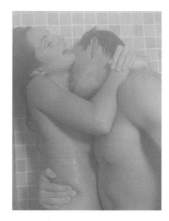

ABOVE AND BELOW | The occasional quickie helps keep the magic alive and can be a timely reminder of exactly how much you love and desire each other.

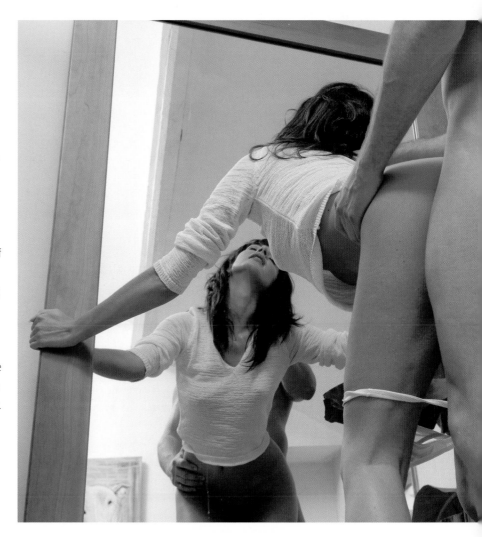

al fresco

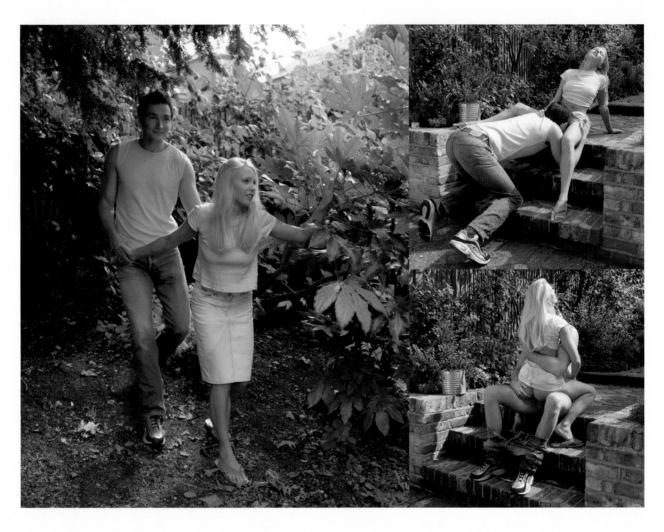

ABOVE | Fresh air and sunshine are natural aphrodisiacs. Whether you are walking in the woods or sitting in your own garden, why not follow your instincts and let nature take its course?

RELEASING YOUR SEXUAL ACTIVITIES from the confines of the four walls of your home and bringing them out into the open air can be a liberating experience. Enjoying each other in the outdoors puts you in touch with nature and makes the experience seem somehow more wholesome, purposeful and natural.

dangerous games

A word of caution here: having sex in public areas is illegal for reasons of public decency and it is vital not to cause offence. This is especially important to bear in mind if you are travelling abroad as some countries have harsh legal penalties. Equally, while some people find the risk – however slight – of

being observed a positive turn-on, this can have precisely the opposite effect on others. As with all sexual activities, coercing an unwilling partner to have *al fresco* sex will sacrifice long-term fulfilment for short-term satisfaction.

There is something about the smell and feel of fresh air that ignites a basic passion in all of us. A long walk on a wintry day, with the wind literally taking the breath from your lungs, instils a sense of vitality, one of the most important ingredients of great sex. The proximity of lush vegetation, in the thick of a tall impressive wood or shaded by bushes and plants of nature's choosing, evokes fundamental animal desires and stirs our visceral energy. Even just strolling with your partner through a meadow, into a wood, along the beach or even to the local park is a wonderful prelude to get you both in the mood, whether you have sex outdoors or not.

basic instinct

The key to having great sex outside is to let nature be your guide and to go with whatever feels right. If the urge is suddenly to whip up your partner's skirt while you kneel before her and give her pleasure, it's doubtful she will complain. Open-air sex heightens the senses and intensifies feelings so that many people feel extra close and united. Being outdoors certainly gives an added dimension to the tried and tested positions that you enjoy in the privacy of your bedroom. Even the staid missionary position seems racy when you are outside. Sitting up, entwined in each other is also great, as you can do this with comparative ease. If you need to be quick, there is no need to remove all of your clothes, especially if the woman is wearing a flowing skirt.

The best place to have *al fresco* sex is in your own garden providing that it has suitably tall surrounding vegetation or a wall to prevent your being spotted by the neighbours. You can either spread out some blankets and pillows and,

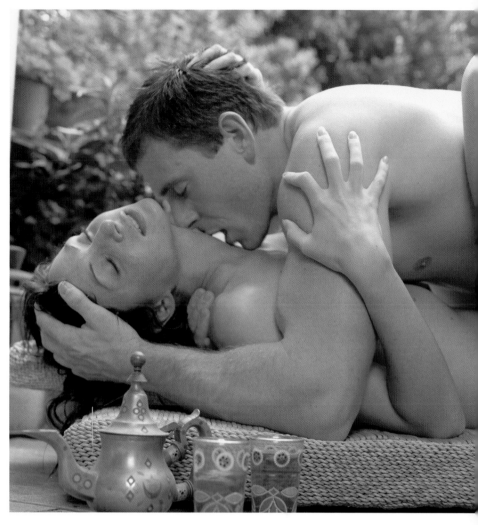

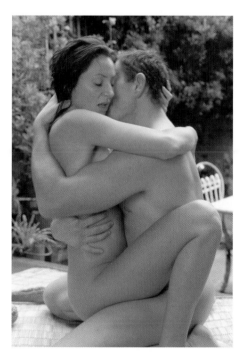

perhaps, some outdoor lights and candles if it is dark, or just go with the moment and get down and dirty in the mud. A garden hammock is a challenge worth taking on. It requires superb co-ordination, but can be done. A swinging garden seat provides a similar momentum with rather less risk of overturning.

Alternatively, if you live in the countryside, then research the area and work out where most people tend to walk and, more importantly, where they don't. Woods are always good, as there are many clearings and concealing bushes to choose from. Places that are harder to get to are usually better. A few things to consider are, how far away you are from a public footpath, where the nearest road is and whether there are any houses nearby. You don't want to end up making love in someone else's back garden.

ABOVE | A quiet cup of tea in the garden could turn into an intense and romantic lovemaking experience.

LEFT | Outdoor sex heightens the senses – touch most of all – and creates a powerful feeling of unity.

sharing sensuality

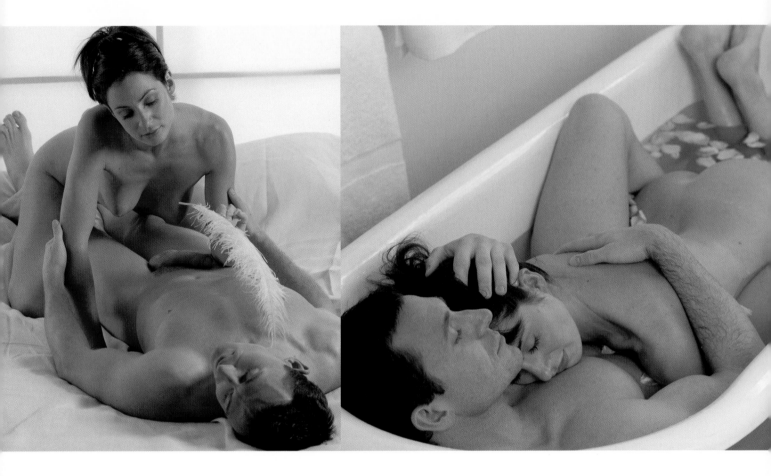

ABOVE | The light touch of a soft feather against bare skin is unbearably erotic.

ABOVE RIGHT | Get yourselves in the mood by sharing a warm, fragrant bath before an erotic session.

SHARING A WARM BATH is a perfect way to begin a massage and an evening of total indulgence and pampering. Many people associate water with relaxation and comfort and it is a wonderfully sensual stimulant. A warm, fragrant bath together is extremely erotic, as you luxuriate in the soft, silky textures of each other's bodies. The skin's responsiveness to touch is enhanced and the water's enveloping properties help you both to feel more united.

no touching

For added eroticism, give your partner a "hands free" massage. Tell your partner to close his or her eyes. The only rule is that you cannot touch one another with any part of your body. If you both have long hair, you can use it to caress one another. Make sure it is clean and smells nice.

Begin by putting your hair over your head and softly and slowly dragging it around your partner's body, starting from the head. You can add to the sensation by softly blowing on their skin at the same time. When you reach the most sensitive areas such as nipples, groin or armpits, allow your hair and breath to linger, gently circling and stroking to build anticipation.

Now try using a feather to caress your partner. Feathers are very sensuous, as the soft, light texture can be used in so many different ways. You can drag it slowly over the skin, following a path of your own choosing, or try a sharper, flicking motion, concentrating on specific areas. Whether you are male or female, being stroked by a feather is a delicious sensation. Make sure that your partner's eyes are tightly closed or that they are blindfolded before you start stroking them –

losing the use of one sense heightens all the others. Ask them to guess what it is you are using. If they guess correctly, reward them by spending extra long on their genital area. If they guess incorrectly, reprimand them by tickling their armpits or nose.

feathering

If you are stroking your man and he becomes aroused, ask him to lie on his back and place the feather between his hard penis and his stomach. Rub it up and down or forwards and backwards. Then get him to open his legs and, as you sit between them, run the feather up from his perineum, over his testicles and along the shaft before going back down again. Vary the sensation, so that on one stroke you keep the feather light, barely touching him, on another you use a firmer, circular motion, and on a third, you sweep it in quick sharp strokes, left and right, up and down.

Use your imagination to find other sensuous textures. Try the contrasting sensations of a bead necklace running over the skin, the softness of a leather glove, the barely there lightness of silk stockings or satin lingerie, the slight roughness of lace or the tactility of fake fur.

Another deliciously erotic sensation is the feel of ice against the skin. Run an ice cube over your lover's body and watch how their nipples harden as you gently circle the cube around them. Gently slide it around their genitals, holding it in your mouth at the same time, so they feel the heat from your breath and the chill from the ice. Be careful around the clitoris, as an ice cube may be too much for some women. Opt instead for running it over her inner labia for a more muffled chill.

Another way to excite the senses is to sprinkle the petals of your lover's favourite flower over their body so that they can luxuriate in the smell and the soft tickle of the velvety texture.

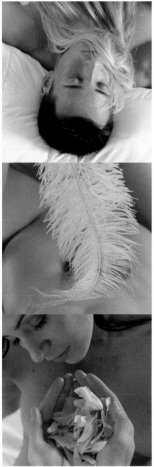

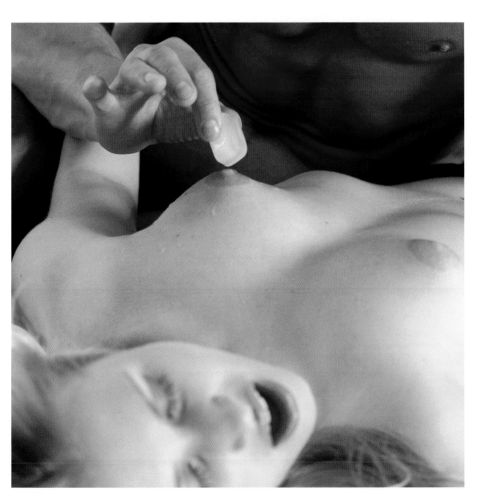

ABOVE TOP | If you have long, silky hair, brush it all over your lover's body for a unique "hands off" massage.

ABOVE CENTRE | Flick the feather over the aroused genitals for the full effect.

ABOVE BOTTOM | Showering your lover with fragrant petals is romantic and sensuous.

LEFT | An icy touch is a thrilling and tantalizing sensation.

erotic massage

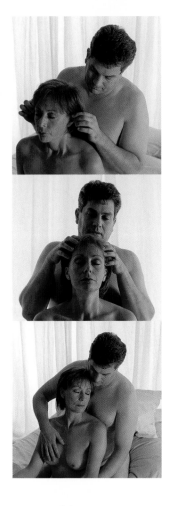

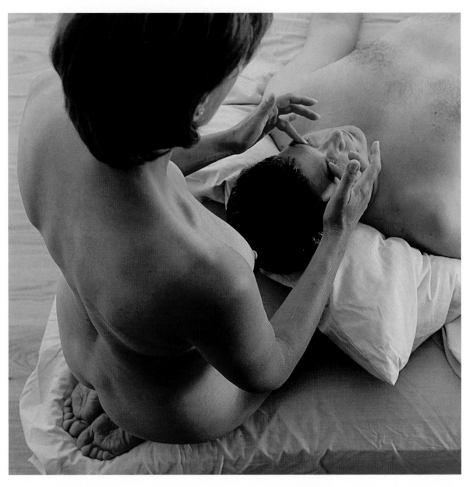

ABOVE TOP | The ears are a powerful erogenous zone – massaging them can be erotic.

ABOVE CENTRE | A head massage is superbly relaxing, helping to release all the day's stress and tension.

ABOVE BOTTOM | You can massage your partner's breasts by kneeling behind her.

ABOVE RIGHT | Massaging the delicate skin of the face feels strangely intimate.

A HEAD MASSAGE is one of the nicest gifts you can give your partner, especially if they have had a hard day, as it releases all tension.

Ask your partner to sit comfortably, while you sit or stand behind. Take off jewellery that might catch on their skin, then place your fingertips on the scalp. Run your open fingers softly through the hair. With quite a firm circular motion, rotate your fingers around the scalp, changing the size of the circles and gradually increasing the pressure. Concentrate on areas such as behind the ears, along the hairline and the base of the skull.

Now concentrate on the forehead, gliding your thumbs from the top of the nose in an arch to the sides of the head and back. Repeat, following the line of the eyebrow, and adapt it by using

small circular strokes with the balls of your thumbs. Next, sweep your thumbs gently down the sides of the nose and across the sinuses, then out towards the cheekbones before repeating.

Cup your hands into a loose fist and support the back of the ears with the side of your first finger, using your thumbs to make small circular motions all around the rims. Then move down to grasp the lobe between the tips of your thumb and index finger and gently pull it down, allowing it to slip through your fingers before repeating.

shoulders

A good place to start a full body massage is the shoulders and back, as these areas often contain the most knots and tight muscles. By easing the tension there, you pave the way for a totally relaxing and sensual full body massage – truly a great act of love.

Ask your partner to lie on their front. Put a small amount of massage oil on your hands and rub them together to warm it. Start at the top of the shoulders with both hands flat on the skin with the neck between them. Run your hands up the back of the neck, then down and along the tops of the shoulders in long sweeping strokes. Repeat with a firmer pressure using your thumbs. Begin to focus on specific areas, gradually increasing the pressure, pressing your thumbs into the muscular areas, using small circular strokes until you can feel the muscles loosening up. Punctuate the more intense circular strokes with the sweeping strokes to add variety and encourage relaxation.

Extend your massage down your partner's back. Place your hands flat on either side of the top of the spine and sweep down to the base. On the upward sweep, apply more pressure by using your body weight. Vary this stroke by sweeping your hands out to the sides using fanning strokes or a harder circular pressure with the heels of your hands. Avoid directly massaging the spine.

breasts

Massaging a woman's breasts is sensual and erotic for both parties. It is best done with the woman lying on her back. You may find it easier to straddle your partner, but do not sit on her. Begin by placing your hands palms down under each breast with your thumbs out to form an "L" shape and the breast cupped in the crook of the "L". Using quite firm pressure, circle your hands upwards and inwards and as they rotate inwards, bring the thumb and index finger together so that they end up lightly pinching the nipples before beginning again. If you want, you can concentrate on one breast, using a similar technique but this time with one hand following the other to complete the circle.

Another technique is to use your fingers and thumbs to pinch the nipple area gently before slowly fanning out your fingers across the breast. Use a light pressure around the nipple and increase the pressure as your fingers span out.

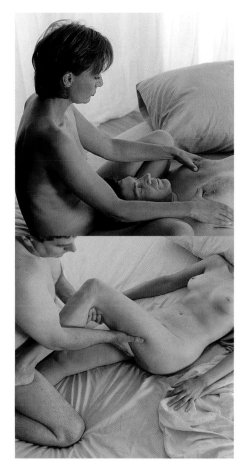

thighs

It is easier to massage the thighs with your partner lying on their back, as they can bend their knees. Cup one hand on the underside of the thigh and the other on the top, just above the knee. Increase the pressure in the tips of your thumbs and fingers as you glide your hands up the length of the thigh and down again. The inner thigh is very sensitive, so vary your strokes from feather-light to harder fanning, using the heel of your hand to give pressure in a constant sweeping motion.

buttocks

Sit at your prone partner's side and softly knead the buttocks with both hands, gradually increasing the pressure. Next, hold your hands above one buttock, keeping them taut, flat, straight and parallel, and use a sharp chopping motion to strike it. Use alternate hands and move up and down the length of the buttock. Then repeat on the other buttock before going back to kneading.

LEFT | Men also enjoy having their chests massaged, using a similar technique to breast massage. As the pectorals are less sensitive, you can use a firmer pressure. Use the balls of your fingers to do small circles on the whole area, but especially the sides and the groove of the armpit.

BELOW LEFT | You can tease your partner when massaging their thighs by lightly brushing your hands "accidentally" over their genitals on the upward stroke, gradually increasing the frequency and pressure of these "accidents".

BELOW | Breasts and buttocks are usually the fleshiest part of the body but need different treatments. The soft vibrations from your hands will also run down to their genitals and fuel their excitement.

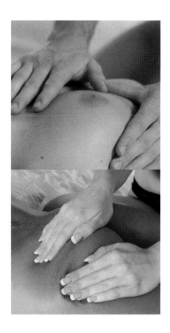

trying something new

BELOW | Nothing ventured, nothing gained. If sex is becoming more like a routine chore than a frenzy of ecstasy, you have the solution almost literally in your own hands. Try something that you have wondered about, but never done before, whether it is rimming, or using a vibrator. Suggest something you enjoyed with a previous partner, but have never done with your current one – you don't have to mention where the idea came from. Think back to the things you used to do together, but now no longer seem to have time for. Stretch your imagination and push the boundaries a little.

TRULY GREAT SEX is usually that which is totally uninhibited, where no holds are barred and where each partner feels completely at ease with their loved one. For many couples, perhaps the majority, this is not the case, even though they may have known their partner for many years, watched their body shape change and feel comfortable and safe in their presence. As time goes on, it gets harder to change, and couples reach a sexual stalemate where they have met their limits. In order to progress, a new level of intimacy must be achieved.

masturbating together

Most people view masturbation as an uninhibited self-pleasuring practice that they have done for many years in private. The idea of masturbating in front of someone else, regardless of how much you may love and trust them, can be daunting.

A good place to begin is to lie between your partner's legs, so they can embrace you, but you do not have the sensation of being watched. Get used to the idea of touching yourself in front of them without worrying about whether you orgasm or not, just to let them see how you like to

touch yourself. Once you are fully comfortable doing this, you can both try masturbating at the same time in front of each other and work on trying to orgasm simultaneously. It is worth noting that watching their partner masturbate is one of the top five male fantasies.

pushing the boundaries

It is precisely because couples feel safe and comfortable together that sex can actually become boring. For some couples, simply letting go of a few inhibitions – and almost everyone has some – can be enough to restore the magic. Try positions and activities that you haven't previously explored, even a little light S&M or anal stimulation.

Don't confront your partner as if this as a challenge or grit your teeth and systematically work through the entire Kama Sutra. However, if you would like to try, say, rimming – licking and kissing the anus – you could both test the water by gently licking and sucking each other's genitals, while stroking and massaging the anal area with your hands. Mirror each other, so that one copies the other. If one chooses to lead, then he or she massages their partner's anus in the way they would like him or her to massage them. The other partner can reciprocate by following this lead – or not, if they don't like it. This is a great way of communicating to each other how you like to be touched in new and sensitive areas.

crossing the line

Trying different positions may not be enough for some highly adventurous couples who feel that they need a more extreme stimulus to enliven a dull sex life and want to push the limits still further. A good place to start is the Internet, as there are plenty of websites catering for all manner of sexual tastes from swingers' clubs to voyeurism. This will give you the opportunity to discover the options, discuss them and form an opinion about whether you both really want to try something

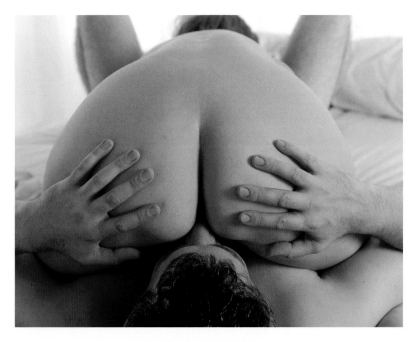

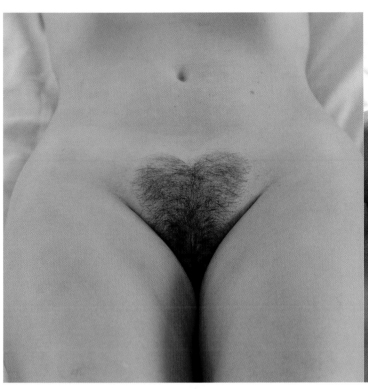

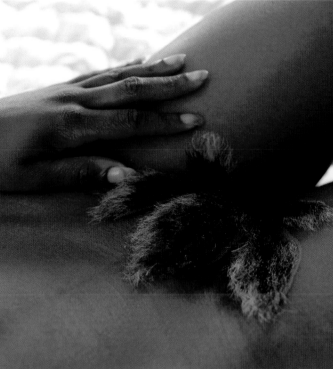

that, perhaps up till now, has just been a fantasy. A trip to a sex shop together would be another way to explore other possibilities, such as bondage and restraint fetishes.

It is important to discuss any activity that might be described as beyond the usual boundaries, especially if it involves other people. The reality of seeing your lover giving pleasure to a third party may be very different from the idea of it and could harm or even ruin a long-term relationship. If you both agree – and it must be both – to proceed with some more off-beat sexual thrills, set some limits about what is and isn't allowed and do some more research to make sure that you will be as safe as possible. If one of you is keen, but the other lukewarm or totally unenthusiastic, keep the idea at fantasy level and watch some blue movies or read porn magazines or raunchy books that will indulge this aspect of your libido.

a bit of fun

Never forget that laughter is a great aphrodisiac and that one reason couples reach a sexual stalemate is that life – and sex – has become boringly predictable and serious.

You might choose to give your partner a surprise the next time he or she sees you naked. There is a whole variety of things that you can do to your pubic hair that will guarantee that they will be equally amused and aroused. Many women wax or shave their pubic hair to keep it trim and tidy, but a variation on this is to shave it into fun patterns or even dye it for the total makeover. The amount of hair you have will determine how much you can do, but as it is pretty much already in a heart shape, it doesn't require too much skill or artistic flair to trim it and sculpt it into that shape, perfect for a Valentine's Day treat. Other shapes could be a star or a cross, or even a chessboard. A beard trimmer is an excellent tool for all genital artists, as it is often thinner and more precise than your average razor.

A merkin is basically a pubic wig or hairpiece, held in place with a special glue. They have been used throughout history for a variety of reasons, including health problems and "public decency", but today people use them for titillating fun. They vary in shape and colour, from fig leaves and flowers to national flags, and are guaranteed to raise more than a smile.

ABOVE LEFT | Heart-shaped pubic hair – the perfect private joke.

ABOVE | A fig-leaf merkin for playing Adam and Eve – watch out for the snake.

BELOW | Masturbating with your partner is deeply intimate.

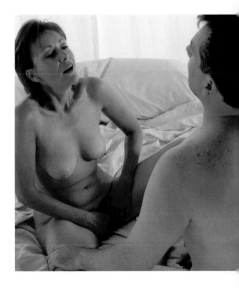

mind games

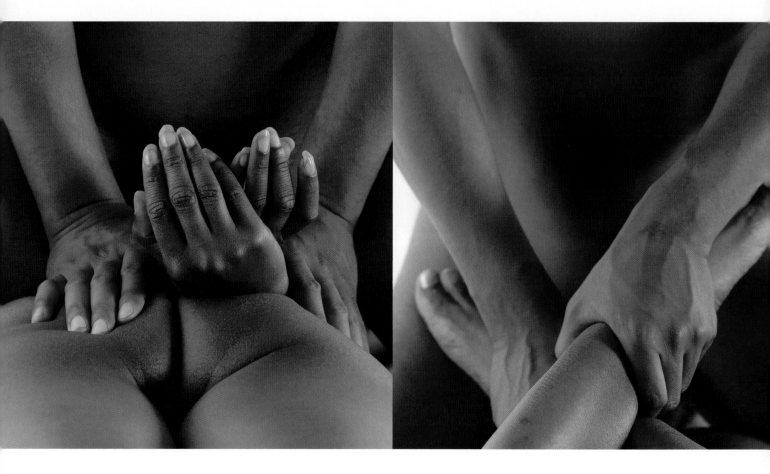

ABOVE | The woman can lie on her front while the man straddles her waist facing her bottom, restraining her hands together behind her back. He can then command her to wrap her restrained hands around his penis as he thrusts in and out of them.

ABOVE RIGHT | Hold your partner's legs bent and they won't be able to escape.

IN LONG-TERM RELATIONSHIPS, fantasies can play an important role in keeping the flames of passion burning. The difficulty often lies in sharing your fantasies with your partner, as many people are afraid of being judged. Most sexual fantasies range from the weird to the subversive and often people fantasize about things during the throes of passion that make them feel uncomfortable when they think of them out of the sexual context, but being unruly is a very human desire. An uninhibited and passionate session of being "naughty" with your partner is an expression of your innermost desires and an act of physical and emotional trust that can enhance a long-term relationship.

Your fantasies are personal and private and it is not necessary to divulge them, but there may be elements of them that you could bring up and explore with your partner. For example, a woman who fantasizes about having sex with two men at the same time could ask her partner to use a dildo or vibrator and double-penetrate her during sex.

restraint
Other common fantasies that couples can explore to spice up a long-term relationship involve restraint. These can range from holding hands or legs down while you stimulate each other, to being physically tied up. One advantage of restraining each other is that it helps you to communicate without actually having to speak. By holding your partner down you are telling them that you don't want them to worry about pleasing you, for now you are going to concentrate on them. All they need do is lie back and enjoy. It is fun to alternate playing the dominant role, in which you take charge of proceedings, with the

submissive role, which takes the pressure off having to please and allows you to relinquish control to your partner's loving hands and kisses.

The great thing about restraint sex games is that they include a frisson of anxiety – which is immensely arousing – but do not have to include pain or fear. Forget the whip-cracking dominatrix and leather mask image of "heavy bondage" (unless that really is your thing) and concentrate on teasing and tantalizing. Loosely tie your partner's wrists and ankles to the bed with silk scarves, stockings or ties so that they are spread-eagled, or invest in a pair of furry handcuffs. Then slowly wreak havoc on their nervous system, by stimulating every inch of their body with your hands, tongue, genitals, a vibrator, a feather – whatever you like – repeatedly drawing back at the last possible moment. Remember, you are in control.

The idea of restraint can be intimidating, as however much you trust and love your partner the feeling and idea of helplessness is not always a pleasant one. To overcome this fear it is sensible to start with a few simple restraint positions such as holding down your partner's hands while covering their body with kisses, or tying your partner to the bed while you perform oral sex on them. Once you are aware of each other's boundaries and how far to take restraint, there are a number of different things that you can do.

Restraint can also be used within role-playing. Whatever your role-play fantasies are, whether it's doctors and nurses or parlour-maid and master, holding each other down or tying each other up can add to the element of excitement.

swinging

Previously known as wife-swapping in the 1950s, swinging has boomed into a lucrative alternative to straight sex. There are now swingers' clubs, swinging festivals and swingers' holidays available for like-minded couples who can go and fulfil their fantasies and desires in a relatively safe environment with other people who share their preferences. Swinging often culminates in group sex, as many swingers find the thrill lies in watching each other making love to different

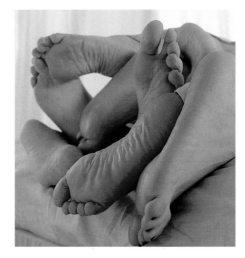

people. There are strict codes of practice and most partners have limits within their relationship as well. For example, usually if one partner does not want to have sex with a certain couple, then they choose not to as a couple, regardless of what the other partner may feel. It is almost always a joint decision. Swingers are usually very open people who are not interested in doing anything against anyone's will. Any couple interested in swinging should consider visiting one of the organized events to talk to other swingers and get more information before they decide whether or not they want to get involved.

see and be seen

Voyeurism and exhibitionism are other sexual activities that give some people a thrill. It is important to point out that watching someone else without his or her knowledge is both illegal and immoral. There is a current trend for car-park parties where people park their car, and allow others to watch them, and sometimes join in, having sex. This is aimed at voyeurs and exhibitionists as it is considered acceptable for other partygoers to wander around the car park, looking through windows and watching what is going on in each car. There are voyeur websites and some sex clubs have voyeuristic viewing rooms.

Obviously, there is an element of risk involved here, and by taking part you are laying yourself open to abuse. Not everyone who takes part in such activities will be as conscientious as you are.

LEFT | Sex in a group is not to everyone's taste, but for some people it can be a great fantasy.

BELOW TOP | Some positions require keeping a firm grip.

BELOW BOTTOM | Try different positions incorporating restraint. For example, he could lie on his back while she gets on top of him and forces him to surrender with her knees.

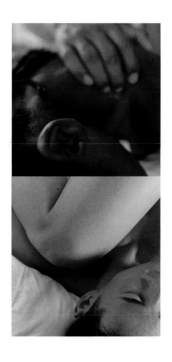

multiple orgasms

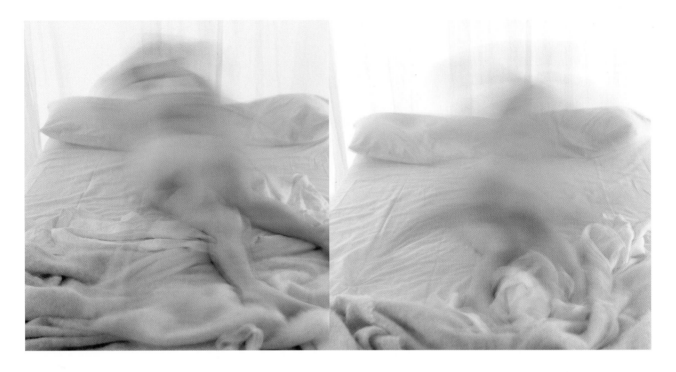

ABOVE AND BELOW | Genital geography can make orgasm during penetrative sex elusive for some women. CAT can solve this and is actually fun for both partners.

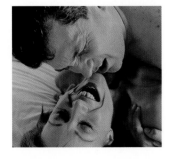

MANY WOMEN HAVE INFREQUENT ORGASMS or no orgasms at all and, over the years, this can take its toll on a relationship. This doesn't necessarily mean that they are not having good sex, but the dynamics of a woman's arousal are quite complex and it doesn't help that the design and position of the clitoris make stimulation somewhat hit or miss. The Coital Alignment Technique (CAT) and the Extended Sexual Orgasm technique (ESO) are two methods that have been designed to overcome some of these difficulties.

coital alignment technique

CAT is a position that has been adapted from the missionary position to greatly increase the likelihood of a woman reaching orgasm during penetrative sex. It is ideal for women who have difficulties achieving orgasm during penetration, although it helps only if these difficulties are technical ones and not psychological.

The clitoris of most women is approximately 2–3cm/¾–1¼in away from the vaginal opening, so clitoral stimulation during penetration is often

sporadic, indirect or totally absent. The difference with CAT is that the man penetrates his partner from a more acute angle, so that his thrusting penis stimulates her clitoris.

Start in the normal missionary position with the man on top, between his partner's spread legs, which she gently bends from the knees. As he enters her, he should lift himself forwards, further up her body, so that his thrusts make contact with her clitoris, keeping his upper body relaxed by leaning either to the left or right to rest part of his weight on the bed. The woman can wrap her legs around her partner's legs, keeping her pelvis stretched so that her ankles lie around the vicinity of his calves.

Another option is for the woman to keep her legs closed while her partner places his legs on the outside of hers. Try both ways to see which one suits you better. The latter may be more beneficial to women with a very sensitive clitoris which does not respond well to direct contact. From here, the couple should begin a light rocking motion back and forth, keeping in rhythm with each other. He should grind and rotate or make figures-of-eight with his pelvis from time to time, as many women respond well to the stimulation of a circular motion around their clitoris.

extended sexual orgasm

ESO was developed by psychiatrist Alan Brauer and psychotherapist Donna Brauer and is designed to help women to extend their orgasms to up to 30 minutes in duration. The woman should begin by training both her mind and body, cleansing herself of any negative barriers or fears she may have about sex by focusing on the enjoyment of sex with her partner. What this means is that she should begin with a couple of weeks of daily pelvic floor muscle workouts and a regular masturbation programme concentrating on learning precisely the types of stimulation she finds the most effective.

ESO is done with the woman lying on her back and her partner between her legs, either kneeling or sitting. As he could be there for anything up to half an hour, he should choose a comfortable position. The man begins by applying lubrication to her entire genital area, massaging everywhere except the clitoris. When the woman begins to move her body to the rhythm of the massage, he should begin slow, rhythmic clitoral stimulation, while she flexes her PC muscles and takes deep breaths. When the first set of orgasmic contractions commences, he should shift stimulation from the clitoris to the vaginal walls, by inserting a couple of fingers, but keeping the rhythm steady and slow. Once she achieves her first orgasm, he should wait for it to subside slightly, but not so long that the contractions stop. He must then continue massaging the vaginal walls slowly and rhythmically and if she feels the contractions subsiding, move back to the clitoris, maintaining the momentum. This should trigger further contractions and so he should move back to the vaginal wall massage, continuing this back and forth movement until the contractions become continuous. Finally, he stimulates both areas at the same time, resulting in wave after wave of continual orgasms.

go again, and again…

For some women it is possible to have more than one orgasm. Some claim that the second or third is less intense, whereas others claim that intensity builds with each one. The techniques for achieving multiple orgasms in women are similar to those described in ESO, where stimulation after the first orgasm continues. Many women find that their clitorises are hypersensitive to touch after orgasm, so instead of stimulating the clitoris directly, her partner should stimulate the surrounding areas until feelings of arousal return.

For men, the multiple orgasm is more difficult to achieve, as many enter a refractory period after ejaculation, which usually means a light snooze. It is believed that men who can separate orgasm and ejaculation are able to experience multiple orgasmic sensations. This is one of the tenets of Tantric and Taoist sex.

In order to achieve this separation, men need to develop strong PC muscles with Kegel exercises. When the man gets to the point of orgasm, he should stop all stimulation and contract his PC muscles, then relax all the muscles of the pelvis and bottom area. He should then resume stimulation and repeat the whole process, before finally squeezing the PC muscles tightly at the point of orgasm. The man should then experience the pleasurable sensations of orgasm without releasing any semen. Anyone with a prostate problem should consult a doctor before trying this.

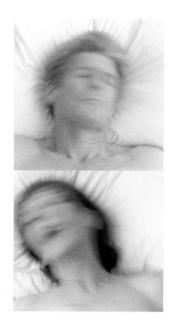

ABOVE AND BELOW | Practising what is known as semen retention, by contracting the PC muscle, enables a man not only to prolong lovemaking and so stimulate his partner to orgasm, but also to have multiple orgasms himself.

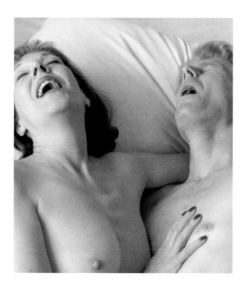

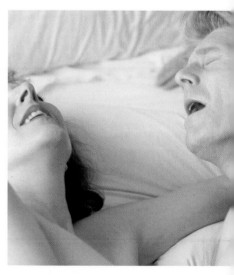

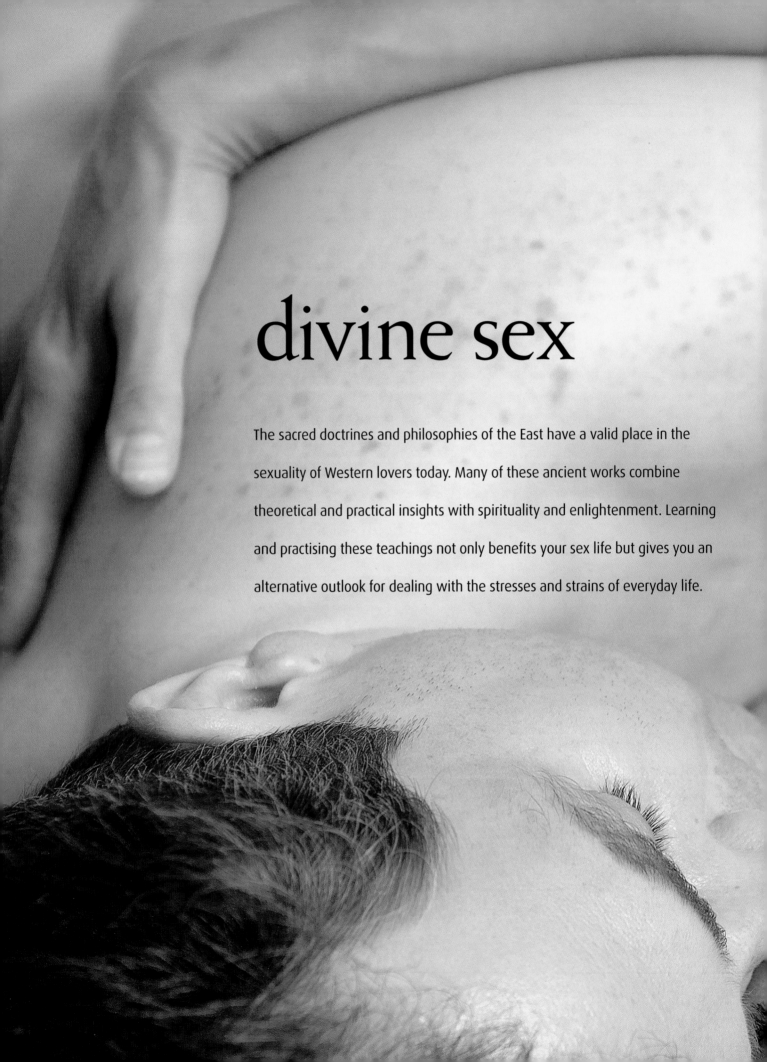

divine sex

The sacred doctrines and philosophies of the East have a valid place in the sexuality of Western lovers today. Many of these ancient works combine theoretical and practical insights with spirituality and enlightenment. Learning and practising these teachings not only benefits your sex life but gives you an alternative outlook for dealing with the stresses and strains of everyday life.

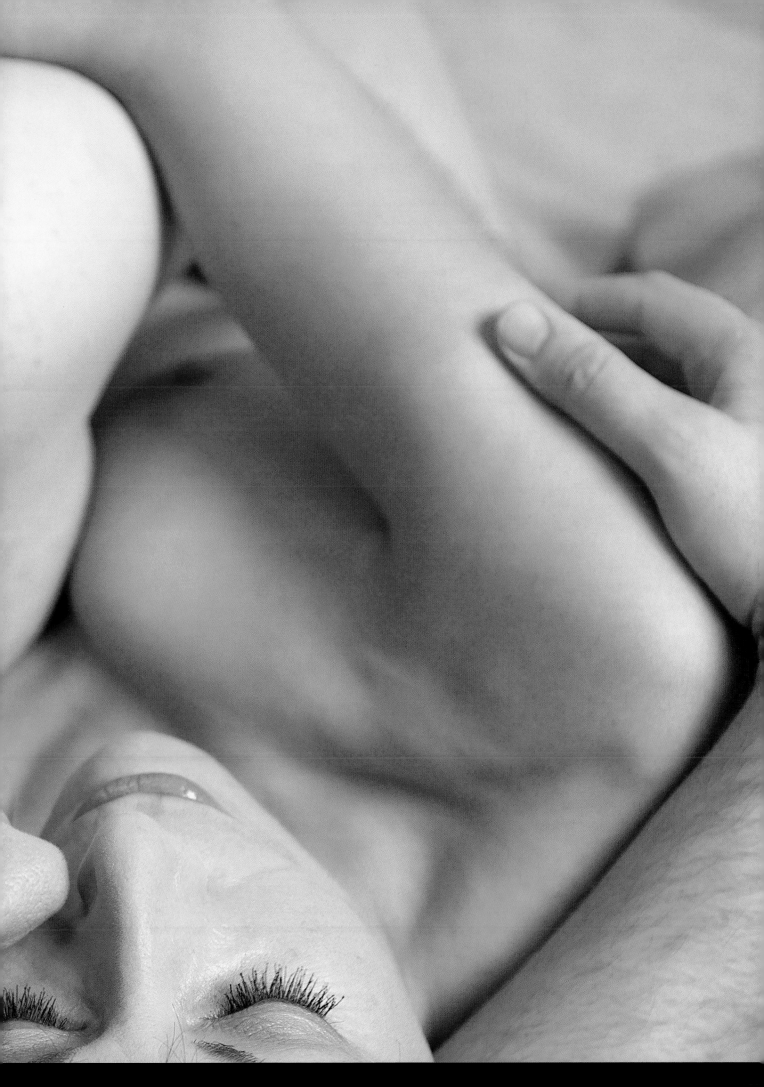

sex and philosophy

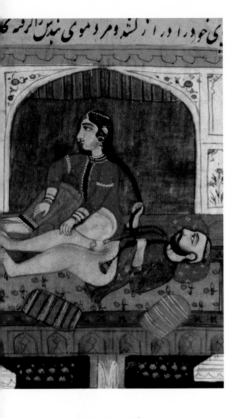

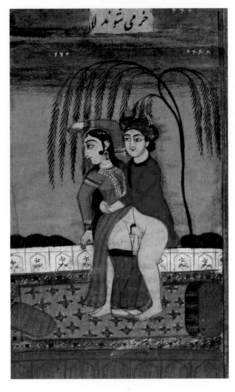

ABOVE | An 18th-century image from the Kama Sutra shows the woman on top while the man pulls her hair.

ABOVE RIGHT | Standing positions were most exalted.

SOME OF THE MOST FAMOUS ancient sex manuals originated in India many hundreds of years ago. The first, the Kama Sutra, is a collection of ancient Hindu writings on sex – known as Vedas – which were themselves based on an earlier oral tradition. It was followed by the Ananga Ranga and later by Tantric philosophy, both of which have used the Kama Sutra in their teachings as a sexual blueprint, adapting the positions and practices.

The Kama Sutra was put together by a student of religion and the divine, Mallanga Vatsayana, sometime between the 1st and 4th centuries AD. In its fearless and uninhibited approach to sexual passion it is more enlightening than the theories of many modern-day erotologists. Due to its explicit content and vivid descriptions of positions and potions intended to enhance lovemaking, it has often been misunderstood in the West as pornographic. In fact, it was intended as a guide to love, detailing courting practices, ways of treating marriage partners and consorts and more.

Over a thousand years after the Kama Sutra, Kalyana Malla's Ananga Ranga appeared. Although Malla used many of the Kama Sutra's sexual positions, embraces and other techniques, the Ananga Ranga had a different aim and content to the Kama Sutra. Whereas the Kama Sutra was associated with love and union, the Ananga Ranga was more orientated towards preventing the separation of husbands and wives and enhancing marriage longevity. Following up on this aim, Kalyana Malla describes the different types of men and women and catalogues their various seats of passion, characteristics and temperaments.

The origins of Tantra are harder to define. The oldest Tantric text seems to be the Buddhist Tantras that date back to around AD 600, but there are Tantric elements in the Vedas. More than a practice or step-by-step guide, Tantra is a philosophy, concerned with spirituality and divine energy, blending sacred sexuality, Eastern philosophy and the teachings of the Kama Sutra. It involves the use of meditation and yoga to master the ultimate goal of dissipating the ego and creating union with the divine energy that is within each of us.

Over the last three thousand years, Eastern cultures have worshipped and respected the power and life force of human sexual nature and recognized the importance of teaching this to the next generation. In the West, our social sexual development has been very different. Although contemporary Western society is more liberal and open than in the past, the arts of seduction, sensuality and wanton abandon have been underdeveloped by comparison with the East. By looking towards the East, we can borrow wisdom and teachings from a long history of enlightened sexual revolutionaries.

kama sutra

Although little is known of the compiler of the Kama Sutra, Mallanga Vatsayana, it is claimed that he was a student Brahmin, involved in the contemplation of the divine. He was probably based in the city of Pataliputra during a period of economic growth and social liberalism.

The Kama Sutra focuses around the three major concepts of Hinduism: *dharma* (the gaining of religious merit or righteousness and responsibility), *artha* (achieving goals, including personal wealth) and *kama* (love and the other sensual pleasures). The theory was that when one had attained these three goals, combining the moral, material and erotic, then one could aspire to acheiving *moksha,* or spiritual liberation.

The Kama Sutra is therefore not solely sexually focused and only a small portion of the text concentrates on the act of sex. In India it became a guide to human relations and interactions. It advises on other aspects of male-female relations such as courtship and marriage, the duties of wife and husband, enhancing beauty and attractiveness, and it provides a variety of recipes and incantations to help with sexual problems and difficulties.

Vatsayana's tone in the Kama Sutra is remarkably unprejudiced and liberal considering the time in which it was written. The emphasis is suggestive as opposed to dictatorial, frequently reminding couples that they should do whatever they feel is right for them at the time. It is a lover's guide, not a lover's law.

The West got wind of the Kama Sutra in the Victorian era, when women were not expected to enjoy sex and men did not therefore require any specific sexual skill or talent to please them. Its Victorian translators, F.F. Arbuthnot and Sir Richard Burton, published the book in English in 1883 for private circulation. It was not until 1963 that the first edition became available to the general public, a hiatus that greatly added to the mystique surrounding the Kama Sutra.

The Kama Sutra is in many ways a direct portal to the period and culture in which it was written. Although much of it is outdated, there are many underlying elements in the Kama Sutra that the Western world can still learn from. The most important of these is the sense of belonging to a civilized society that takes the pleasures of the mind and body extremely seriously.

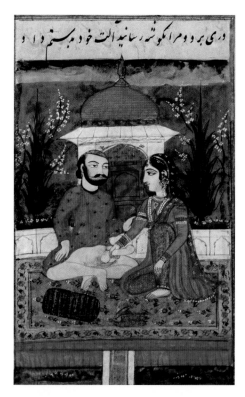

LEFT | In this 18th-century illustration, the woman is manipulating the lingham, or penis, of her partner.

BELOW | Illustrations of the Kama Sutra are often set in beautiful palaces, here complete with flowers, hand-woven rug and hookah.

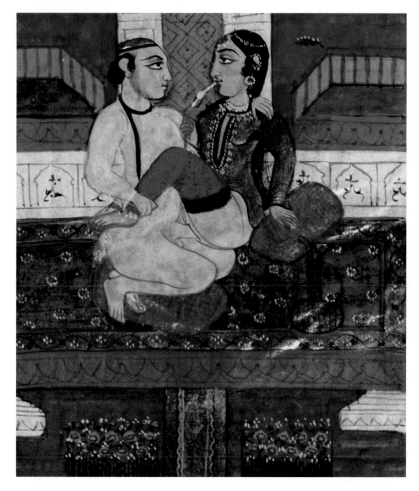

a modern kama sutra

THE KAMA SUTRA isn't just a list of exotic positions for sex. It describes in great detail the delicacy of foreplay and the importance of both parties being satisfied sexually, and also that they should share time together as a couple after congress.

the work of the man

In the Kama Sutra, the "work of the man" denotes any action that the man must do in order to give pleasure to the woman. Vatsayana suggests that when a man and a woman first come together, they begin by sitting on the bed talking about non-sexual topics and encourage each other to drink wine. While the woman is lying on the man's bed, engrossed by his captivating conversation, the man should loosen her undergarments and "overwhelm her" with kisses if she starts to protest.

When he becomes erect it is suggested that he should begin gently touching her with his hands. If she is shy or it is the first time they have had sex together, he should begin by placing his hands between her thighs. He should also caress her breasts, neck and armpits with his hands.

modern interpretation

The contemporary message of the concept of "the work of the man" is about the importance of foreplay. Take time to seduce each other in bed with words and actions and some good wine. The woman does not have to be passive; both should luxuriate in the sensuality of each other's body before actually having intercourse.

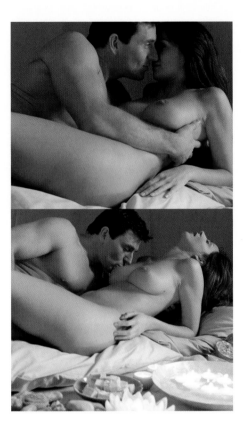

satisfying a woman

During sex, the man should concentrate on pressing the parts of the woman's body "on which she turns her eyes". Signs that a woman is enjoying herself are that she will turn (roll or close) her eyes, will become less shy and will press herself towards him to keep their sex organs as closely united as possible. When the woman shakes her hands, prevents the man from getting up, bites or kicks him, or continues writhing after he has orgasmed, it signifies that she is aroused and requires more satisfaction.

modern interpretation

It is interesting that Indian culture was so aware of the sexual needs of women at a time when the Western world seemed completely oblivious of them. Male reading of the body movements of women during intercourse allows you both to remain at the same tempo. If the man comes before his partner and ignores her need for sexual fulfilment he will invariably leave her frustrated.

sanskrit

The Kama Sutra was written in Sanskrit, the ancient and sacred language of India, in which Hindu literature from the Vedas downwards was composed.

Yoni is the Sanskrit word for the female genitalia, or vulva. The yoni is an object of veneration among Hindus as it is seen as a holy symbol of the goddess Shakti.

Lingham is the Sanskrit word for the phallus, which is worshipped among Hindus as a symbol of the god Shiva.

ABOVE RIGHT | The Kama Sutra was enlightened in its belief in foreplay and recommends that the man should begin by rubbing the woman's yoni with his fingers until aroused.

RIGHT | The woman can clutch the man, pulling him into her body, and demonstrating her physical pleasure.

the end of congress

After sex, the two lovers must show modesty by not looking at each other and by going separately to the bathroom. They should eat betel leaves and the man should anoint the woman's body with sandalwood. He then must embrace her with his left arm and hold a cup in his right, from which he should encourage her to drink.

Together they should eat sweetmeats, soup, mango juice or lemon juice mixed with sugar, anything that is sweet and pure. The couple should then sit outside on a balcony and enjoy the moonlight, with her lying in his lap as they talk. As they gaze at the night sky he should show her the different constellations of stars and planets.

modern interpretation

Don't panic, most women today do not consider an astronomy lesson an essential post-coital activity, although if you do know a bit about stars and planets it can be romantic to share it. Following the above advice is actually a perfect way of spending time together after you have had sex. Enjoy these moments – share a drink, massage one another, feed each other with confectionery, fruit or have a light meal, before cuddling up together for a chat. Stargazing is optional.

the elephant woman

A Hastini, or elephant woman, is a woman with a large vagina. According to Vatsayana, if a man is unable to satisfy a Hastini, various forms of congress are recommended where the woman presses her thighs together, thus increasing the sensations for both parties.

An alternative is to use an apadravyas, an instrument put around or on the penis to make it longer or thicker. Apadravyas should be made of gold, silver, copper, iron, ivory, buffalo horn, various kinds of wood, tin or lead and should be cool and well fitted.

modern interpretation

Although it is not terribly polite to refer to women with large vaginas as elephant women, it is a fact of nature that with age and after childbirth, the vagina may lose some of its tightness. Pelvic floor and Kegel exercises do help to keep the vagina tight but for some women, it is just the way they are. Luckily for contemporary lovers, men no longer need to strap a buffalo horn to their genitals in order to satisfy a woman who has lost her grip. Today there is a wide range of gadgets that will satisfy all shapes and sizes and incorporating them into your sex lives can be great fun.

BELOW LEFT | At the end of congress, sharing some jasmine or mint tea with some sweet food is a marvellous way to bask in the afterglow of sex.

BELOW | Turkish delight is a modern equivalent to Vatsayana's "sweetmeats".

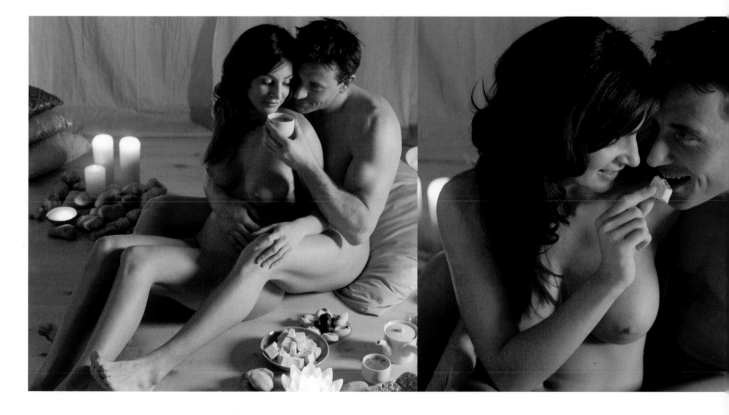

ananga ranga

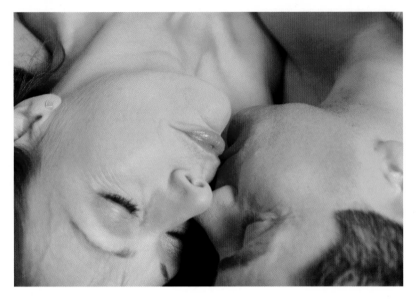

ABOVE AND BELOW |
Closeness continues to be important in a long-term relationship. The Ananga Ranga sought to increase intimacy and rid marriages of any stagnation.

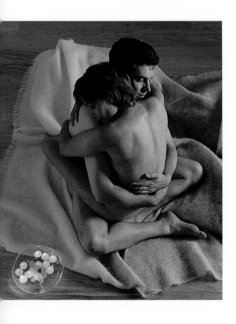

INDIAN LOVE SAGE KALYANA MALLA wrote the Ananga Ranga during the 16th century. It was aimed at keeping husbands and wives from separating when their relationship went wrong. Like the Kama Sutra, the book was translated into English in the late 1800s, but it was not made extensively available until the 1960s as it was considered too racy.

The Ananga Ranga aimed to define more clearly the distinction between monotony and monogamy, releasing one from the other, and relieving the tedium of marriage. Malla believed that the chief reason that husbands go off with other women, and wives with other men, is that sex becomes boring and mundane: "the monotony which follows possession". He wrote a long treatise of erotic work, which incorporated the much older Kama Sutra, describing a multitude of ways of kissing, embracing and sexual positions.

"Fully understanding the way in which such quarrels arise, I have in this book shown how the husband, by varying the enjoyment of his wife, may live with her as with thirty-two different women, ever varying the enjoyment of her, and rendering satiety impossible." The Ananga Ranga seeks to help couples to renew their desire for sex,

which in turn helps them to re-establish strong bonds, both of friendship and love. Although sex is clearly important to all loving relationships, Malla removes the emphasis from sex and argues instead that this should be the end result of all the teachings and techniques that can be introduced to the relationship via the Ananga Ranga. It defines the different types of men and women and their needs, what kind of sex they enjoy and how to hold each other physically, mentally and emotionally.

The contemporary significance of the Ananga Ranga lies in its insistence upon the importance of maintaining passion in long-term relationships and its practical suggestions for rejuvenating stagnant patterns. Despite its antiquity, the concepts and practices set out in the Ananga Ranga are relatively new to the West. By combining the elements of Eastern magic and mystery with what we already know, we can begin to understand how and why problems have arisen in our relationships and begin to take positive steps towards healing wounds and strengthening bonds.

thirty-two lovers

The Ananga Ranga differs from the Kama Sutra in its recognition that the ability to maintain erotic interest in an exclusive monogamous relationship is not simple.

The book defines the difference between intimacy and familiarity and encourages sexual partners to break down the patterns of laziness that are bred from familiarity and to reinvent and renew the possibilities of sustained eroticism that can be derived from true intimacy. It teaches couples to use their minds and imaginations to achieve a more sophisticated level of eroticism and aims to teach lovers to experience their partner as if they were thirty-two different lovers.

embracing techniques

THE ANANGA RANGA'S CHAPTER on the "treating of external enjoyments" concentrates on the importance of various preliminaries that should precede sex and internal enjoyment. These include the various types of kissing and embracing, biting, scratching and hair pulling. These acts, according to Malla, "affect the senses and divert the mind from coyness and coldness." Foreplay is an essential part of all sexual encounters, as it helps to relax and acquaint the partners with each other's bodies and erogenous zones, allowing both to reach the same levels of excitement before penetration.

Malla recommends these techniques for embracing in relationships where cuddling has ceased to be spontaneous. Touching is one of the mutually satisfying ways for men and women to show their affection for each other – not just when they are going to have sex, but at other times as well. The types of pressure to be used are described as pressing, touching, piercing and rubbing. Once tried, these techniques might arouse interest in further contact, or can just be enjoyed in their own right.

vrikshadhirudha

This is often referred to as the embrace that simulates climbing a tree. The woman places one foot on the man's foot and raises her other leg, resting her foot upon his thigh. She puts her arms around his back and holds him tightly.

modern interpretation

With the woman's legs parted in this fashion, and the man's hands relatively free, this embrace gives the man good access to the woman's breasts and genitals for light stroking and caressing, while she showers him with passionate kisses.

tila-tandula

The man and woman stand in front of each other and hold each other closely around the waist. Then, being careful to remain still, he should allow

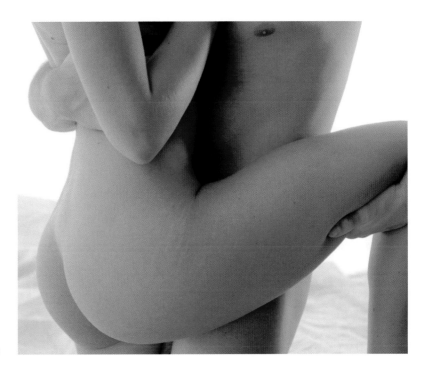

his penis to come into contact with her vagina, with only the veil of her skirt between the two. They should remain like this for a time.

modern interpretation

This embrace is best achieved if the woman is wearing loose clothing made of soft fabric, as the sensation of the material against both the man's and the woman's private parts will add to the experience. It may be hard to remain like this for a long time, as the sensation of each other's genitals in such close proximity is arousing, and can be too much for some.

urupaguha

The man and woman stand in front of each other and he places her closed legs between his own, so that his inside thigh touches her outside thigh. As with all the embraces, the couple should also experiment with kissing at the same time.

modern interpretation

This is an especially good embrace if the man is taller than the woman. The squeezing of her thighs provides gentle stimulation of her clitoris and his genitals are pressed against her.

ABOVE | Climbing a tree – it is as if the woman is trying to reach up for a kiss.

BELOW | Embracing doesn't have to be done by the book – if you are lucky it will happen spontaneously.

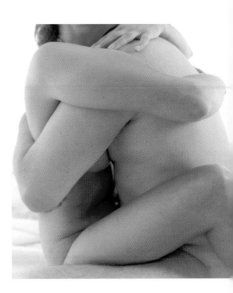

kissing techniques

THE ANANGA RANGA described osculations, or kissing, as particular styles to be studied and which were to be practised with the embracing techniques. "There are seven places highly proper for osculation, in fact, where all the world kisses." These are the lower lip, both the eyes, both cheeks, the head, the mouth, the breasts and lastly, the shoulders. Of course there is no reason why you should stop there.

nlita kissing

When the woman is angry, the man should forcibly cover her lips with his own and continue until her anger has subsided.

modern interpretation

This type of kissing can be a fantastic means of ending an argument in which there is simply nothing more that can be said. Couples who have been together for a long time often find themselves arguing over petty annoyances.

These arguments are usually cyclical in content and it can be hard to walk away or end the quarrel. A kiss such as this requires no words. It says, "Let's forget this, we are arguing over trivia and I love you."

sphrita kissing

The woman leans in to kiss her partner, who kisses her lower lip while she jerks her mouth away without returning the kiss.

modern interpretation

This is a playful, teasing kiss. When you move in to kiss your partner, allow him or her a taste of your lower lip before withdrawing and not allowing the kiss to continue. This is a great one to do in a quiet corner in the company of others. It tells your partner that you are feeling playful and frisky, but that he or she will have to wait until you decide when play will commence. It guarantees anticipation and excitement in your partner and is a seductive means of communicating without words.

BELOW | Nlita kissing – a great way of putting a stop to petty squabbles.

BELOW RIGHT | The teasing sphrita kiss can be initiated by either partner.

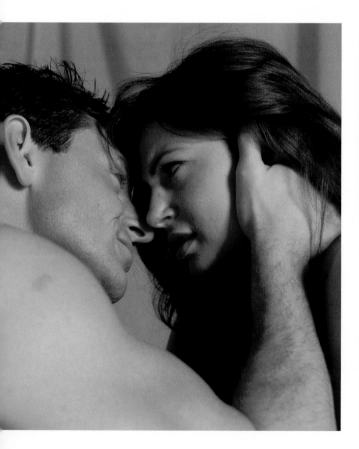

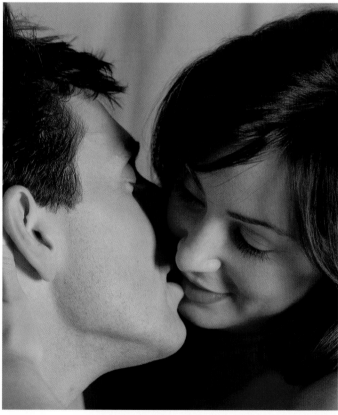

ghatika kissing

The man covers his partner's eyes with his hands and closes his own eyes before thrusting his tongue into his partner's mouth, moving it to and fro using a slow, pleasant motion that suggests another form of enjoyment.

modern interpretation

By removing one sense, in this case sight, the partners' bodies become more attuned to other sensations. In this case, sex is simulated with the mouth, building anticipation about how each will pleasure the other genitally. It is a provocative yet romantic method of kissing, ideal as a precursory invitation to a night of sensational sexual activity.

uttaroshtha

The man gently bites and nibbles his partner's lower lip while the woman reciprocates on his upper lip, then they swap over, both exciting themselves to the height of passion.

modern interpretation

This is like foreplay for kissing. With each other's mouths, the partners tease the nerve endings, so that by the time they begin a more passionate kiss, including tongues, all the sensory organs in the area will be in overdrive, and aroused beyond words.

pratibodha

When one partner is sleeping the other should fix their lips over their sleeping partner's lips, and gradually increase the pressure until sleep turns into desire.

modern interpretation

This kiss ignites passion first thing in the morning, and there is, after all, no better way to begin the day. Begin by gently kissing your partner, gradually increasing the pressure, sucking on his or her lips until they wake up.

tiryak kissing

The man places his hand beneath the woman's chin, and raises it, until he has made her face look up to the sky; then he takes her lower lip between his teeth, gently biting and chewing it.

modern interpretation

It would feel wonderful for a woman to surrender to this gently forceful kiss from a man.

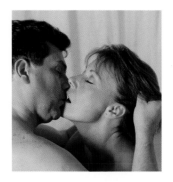

ABOVE | Here, playfully nibbling the lip is combined with pulling the hair.

BELOW LEFT | Ghatika kissing – this is a very suggestive way to arouse your partner's desire for more.

BELOW | Uttaroshtha kissing – he bites her lip, and she bites his; just be sure not to bite too hard...

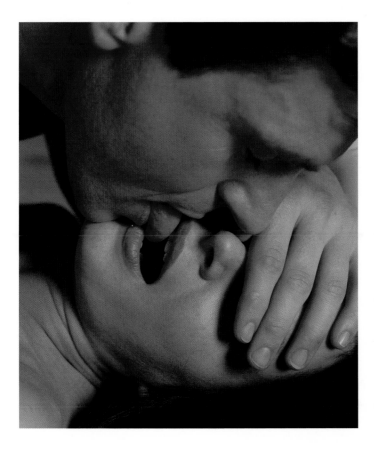

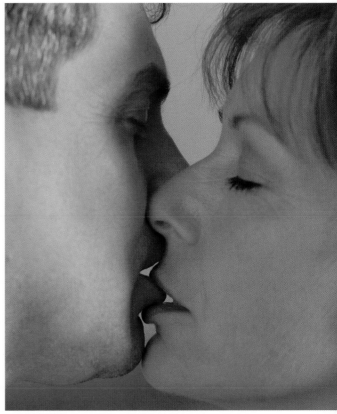

scratching, biting and hair pulling

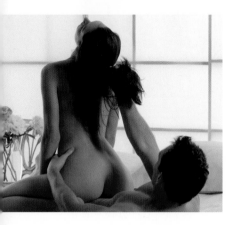

SCRATCHING AND BITING are, both the Ananga Ranga and the Kama Sutra suggest, to be tried only when love becomes intense. Description is given of the preferred, clean state of nails and teeth, and the willingness of both parties, before commencing.

scratching

The Ananga Ranga defines specific times when this type of sex play is advisable. Some examples include: when one partner is about to go away for a long period of time, or when both are "excited with desire of congress." It appears to have been done as a form of remembrance, so that when they are separated there will be a mark on the body to remind them of each other.

ABOVE | The ancient texts were witness to the effect that a woman's hair can have on a man.

BELOW | Light scratching can be extremely erotic if both partners are willing.

churit-nakhadana – gentle scratches

This involves the light scratching of the nails around the cheek, lower lip and breasts. The scratching should be light enough that it leaves no marks.

modern interpretation

The scratching described here is so light that it is more of a caress. The soft use of nails, however, indicates greater passion and energy than a more delicate touch.

the peacock's foot

For this specialist imprint the thumb is placed on the nipple and four fingers are spread adjacent to this on the breast. The nails are dug in to leave an indentation similar to that of a peacock footprint.

modern interpretation

Most women love to have their breasts caressed and squeezed during lovemaking. The preferred pressure and sensation is individual to each woman, with some having very sensitive breasts, especially around menstruation. Before digging your nails into your partner's breasts it is advisable to find out how much stimulation she prefers.

anvartha-nakhadana – to remember

Marks or scratches three deep are made by the first three fingers on the woman's back, breasts or genitals. It is most commonly done as a token of remembrance before the man leaves to go abroad.

modern interpretation

Many men and women really enjoy scratching if it is done correctly, as it is a form of sensual massage and can be very relaxing. Remember to be gentle and do not do anything that may cause pain. As with all these techniques, keep your nails smooth, clean and reasonably short.

biting

The Ananga Ranga suggests that biting should be done in similar places to scratching but lovers should avoid the eyes, upper lip and tongue. It also suggests that the pressure should be increased until the recipient protests, after which enough has been done. Neither party will be in particular favour if they bite the other too hard; soft nibbling is more advisable. Take cues from each other, rising to a passionate moment with appropriate strength, and a lighter touch when called for.

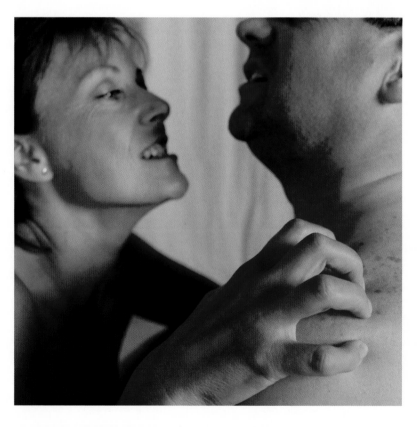

uchun-dashana – biting

This is the generic term to describe biting any part of the woman's lips or cheeks.

modern interpretation

Gently nibbling around each other's faces can be very sensual. Be careful around the bony areas like the cheeks, as they bruise easily. The lips should be handled with care too, as they are only protected by a thin layer of skin.

bindhu-dashana – teeth marks

This is the mark left by the man's two front teeth on the woman's lower lip.

modern interpretation

The lower lip is very supple and elastic and gentle sucking and nibbling on it is very pleasurable. In the days when the Ananga Ranga was written it was probably pretty acceptable for women to bear the marks of their husband's desire. Any imprint of passion today is reminiscent of the adolescent love bite, and not particularly desirable, so facial markings should be avoided.

kolacharcha – on departing

These are the deep, lasting marks left on the woman's body in the heat of passion and the grief of departure when her husband is going away.

modern interpretation

The fleshier parts of the body such as the thighs and buttocks can withstand more pain than the more sensitive areas around the face. They also have the added advantage of being hidden by clothing. Biting each other is a common outlet of sexual energy when in the throes of orgasm and many people, male and female, claim that they have been surprised at the depth of a bite afterwards. Many people enjoy sharp pain at the height of passion to enhance the powerful shudders of pleasure that they experience during orgasm.

hair pulling

Softly pulling the hair of a woman, states the Ananga Ranga, is a good method of kindling a lasting desire.

samahastakakeshagrahana – stroking

The man strokes his partner's hair between the palms of his hands, at the same time kissing her with passion.

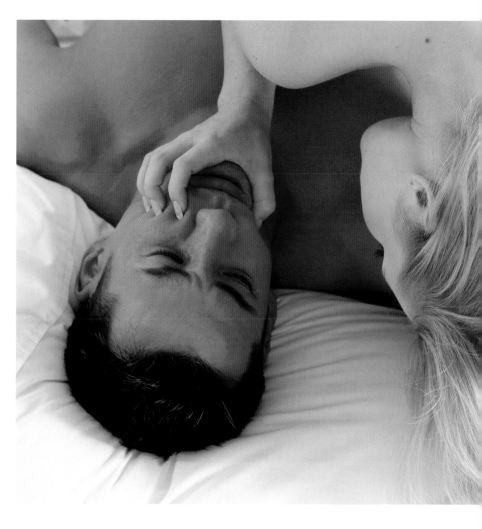

modern interpretation

Gentle pulling and playing with a woman's hair is very erotic and sensual. When pulling hair, make sure you get a good handful, as pulling at a small number of hairs can be very painful. Why not take this a stage further and gently pull tufts of each other's pubic hair – sure to bring each other to a state of excitement.

kamavatansakeshagrahana – pulling

This is done during sexual intercourse, when each partner grabs the other's hair above the ears as they kiss passionately.

modern interpretation

This type of hair pulling is ideal in the throes of passion when the body's touch sensors are dulled by the other erotic sensations that are flowing around. Stroking and massaging this area, including the temples, can be very seductive, especially if you whisper in each other's ears at the same time.

ABOVE | Churit-nakhadana – light scratching around the face – shouldn't leave a mark.

BELOW | He grabs her hair in kamavatansakeshagrahana.

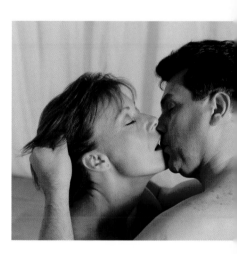

ananga ranga positions

MANY OF THE SEXUAL POSITIONS in the Ananga Ranga were adapted by Malla from the original work of Vatsayana's Kama Sutra. However, Malla's text was written in a very different social climate, where extramarital sex was frowned upon, so the emphasis is on variety with one partner.

the crab embrace

The man and woman lie on their sides facing each other. The man enters the woman and lies between her legs. One of her legs passes over his body (at about the level of his navel) while the other remains beneath his legs.

modern interpretation

The position provides deep penetration and increased friction. The man's movement is limited although the woman has more freedom. This position may be good when one partner is tired but both are still passionate.

kama's wheel

The man sits with his legs outstretched. The woman lowers herself on to his penis, facing him. She also extends her legs. He then stretches his arms out along either side of her body to support her. This forms the wheel-like figure for which this position is named.

modern interpretation

It is said that this position combines sex and meditation to create a higher level of awareness. It is meant to help the partners to obtain a balance of mind that is clear, calm and happy.

the ascending position

The man lies on his back while the woman sits cross-legged upon his thighs. The woman grasps his penis and inserts it into her, moving her waist backward and forward as they make love.

BELOW TOP | Kama's wheel – this is a great transitional position. Try it after ascending or before the placid embrace.

BELOW BOTTOM | The ascending position – this posture can give added satisfaction to the woman.

BELOW RIGHT | The crab embrace, lying side by side, enables plenty of physical contact along the body.

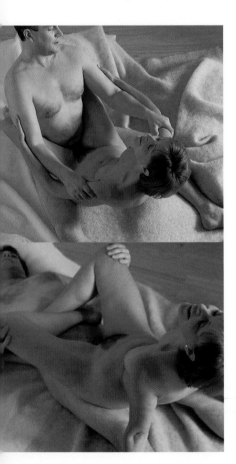

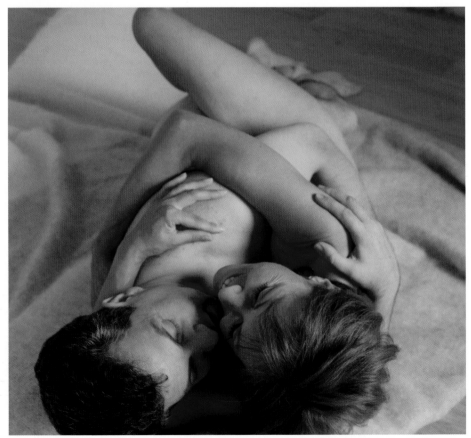

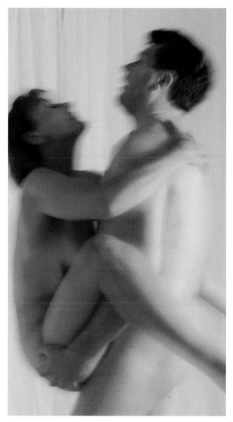

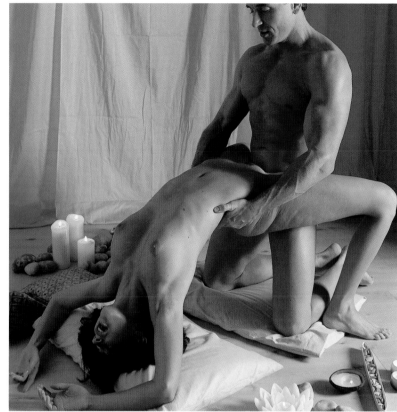

modern interpretation

The woman on top can control the movements and depth of penetration. By moving herself forward and back, her clitoris also receives stimulation from the gentle rubbing action against her partner's body. This is recommended for women who have not found satisfaction in other positions.

suspended congress

Both partners stand opposite one another. The man passes two arms under his partner's knees, supporting her by gripping her inner elbow or her bottom. He then raises her waist high and penetrates her while she clasps her hands around his neck.

modern interpretation

This one could be tricky, as its success depends on many factors such as the strength of the man, the weight of the woman, and the height of them both. It may be easier if the woman gets on a chair first, so that the man does not have to lift her from the ground and risk back injury. It may also help to be near a wall or rail to maintain balance. Good luck!

placid embrace

The man kneels and raises his partner to him by grasping her around the waist so that her head falls towards the floor. She in turn wraps her legs about his middle and lets her head fall freely.

modern interpretation

This position allows the woman to retain some control – by extending and flexing the grip of her legs she can draw her partner closer. Hanging with the head upside-down can also contribute a feeling of ecstasy and otherworldliness. Try this after kama's wheel.

ABOVE LEFT | Suspended congress – this one isn't for you if you have a bad back.

ABOVE | The placid embrace allows the woman to let herself go completely.

BELOW | You may have tried the crab embrace before without realizing it.

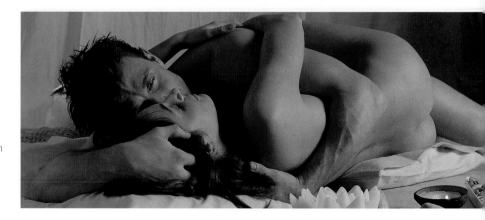

the art of tantric sex

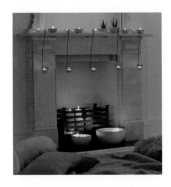

ABOVE | Create a harmonious environment to share.

BELOW | Place your hand on your lover's heart so you can merge together.

BELOW RIGHT | Meditate with your partner, concentrating on each chakra in turn.

TANTRA FOCUSES on honouring and respecting your partner as the other half of yourself. Although Tantrists believe that sex is a divine gift that should be celebrated, Tantra is not a religion but a tradition, which can be practised by people of any faith or by non-religious people.

The word Tantra is derived from the Indian Sanskrit meaning, "liberation through expression". Based on early Hindu and Buddhist teachings, or tantras, Tantra unites elements of meditation, yoga and worship to provide practitioners with a more wholesome and intense sexual experience.

Tantra has many dimensions that can take years of study to fully appreciate. This does not mean, however, that people interested in Tantric sex must immerse themselves in study. Instead, it is perfectly valid to take some elements of Tantra and incorporate them into existing sex lives.

In Tantric sex the vagina becomes a sacred space (yoni) and the penis (or lingham) is a "wand of light". Kundalini denotes the life force and sexual energy that flows between sexual partners as they make love. Breathing and visualization exercises help to harmonize this energy. Tantric sex takes the emphasis away from the physicality of the orgasm and concentrates more on spirituality, intimacy and connection. Men are often taught to suppress their orgasm, a Tantric skill known as maithuna, in order to devote their attention to the woman's sexual pleasure. If this all sounds rather pointless from the male perspective, it is worth remembering that once it is mastered, men reap the rewards, keeping sexually active for anything up to an hour with the promise of increased orgasm when it comes. It can also increase the chance of multiple orgasms for their partner and enable the man to "virtually experience" their lover's orgasm as well as their own.

tantra western style

Tantra cannot cure a failing relationship but it's a good prescription for a loving respectful relationship that has become a bit dull. Most people would prefer to tackle the problem of bedroom boredom rather than bailing out of a relationship. According to Tantra, boredom sets in when people make love with only their genitals, not their hearts and minds.

A couple should begin Tantric lovemaking with an idea of what they want and, more importantly, the genuine desire to give their partner what he or

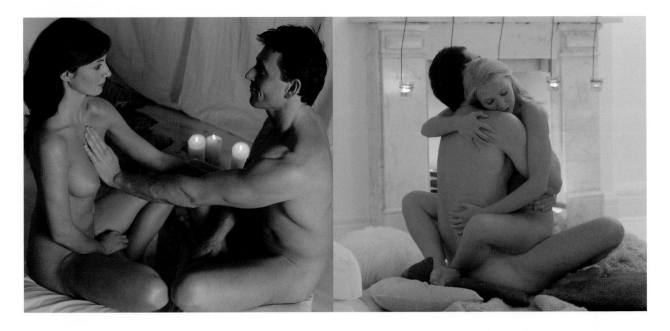

she wants. Tantric sex has no time limit: it can last minutes or hours, and it gives you and your partner the freedom and opportunity to explore each other's bodies and pleasure zones.

Much of Tantric lovemaking involves ritualistic foreplay that excites all the senses. Massage and the use of aromatherapy oils stimulate the senses of smell and touch. By caressing each other slowly and languidly the scene is set for a relaxed session of lovemaking, allowing time to explore each other's bodies and become more comfortable with each other's nudity.

meditation and breathing

Meditation in Tantra is an important principle, as it allows couples to move away from frantic passion, and emphasize tranquillity and harmony.

Dedicate an area for meditation and Tantric lovemaking and set aside a specific portion of uninterrupted time for you to either meditate alone, or with your partner. Make sure that the area is calm and warm, close the curtains, remove distractions, use aromatherapy fragrances such as cedarwood or frankincense, and light some scented candles to add to the atmosphere.

Begin by sitting on the floor with your legs crossed, back straight and hands resting in your lap. Ensure that you are comfortable before closing your eyes and focusing on your breathing. Breathe in through your nose and out through your mouth and become conscious of the soft rise and fall of your diaphragm with each breath. Try to concentrate on your breathing, and every time your mind wanders gently bring it back to your breath. With practice, meditation will create peace and tranquillity and leave you feeling refreshed and calm. Your meditation sessions will become longer, provided you remember to keep patient and relaxed.

tantra to share

Sit in front of each other and look each other in the eye as you place your hands on each other's hearts. As you breathe out, imagine that you are breathing the energy from your heart into your partner's heart. As you breathe in, imagine you are inhaling their energy into your heart. The physical

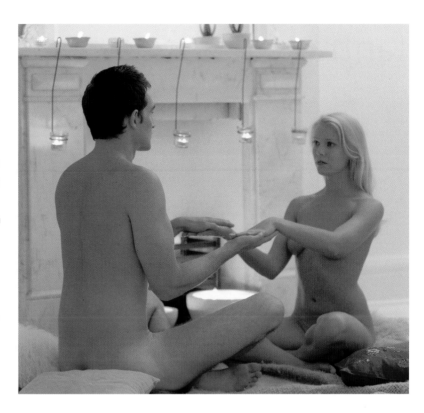

connection allows a circuit of energy to pass between you, so that energy flows from your heart, through your body to your partner's heart, and vice versa. Once you feel comfortable, begin alternating your breathing pattern with your partner's so that as they breathe in, you breathe out and so on. This should cause the energy to circulate evenly and harmoniously between you.

Sit before each other again, but this time merge your energy by placing your palms together, creating an electrical circuit. You can continue with the same breathing techniques or try chakra meditation, in which you concentrate on each chakra, breathing energy into each for two or three minutes. Begin at the base chakra and move up towards the crown, opening up each energy centre as you go. This may take some practice as each of you may require a different amount of time on each chakra, but be patient and before long both your sets of chakras will become harmonized with each other.

Don't be afraid to laugh! The point of this is not to reinvent you as Tantric gurus but to bring you closer together. Collapsing in giggles will not detach you from the spirit of what you are trying to achieve.

ABOVE | Create a circuit of energy between you – merge together for 15 minutes, allowing your breathing to synchronize naturally.

BELOW | A calming and private space in which to meditate will enable you to concentrate and not be distracted by external elements.

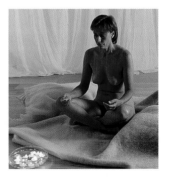

tantra lying down

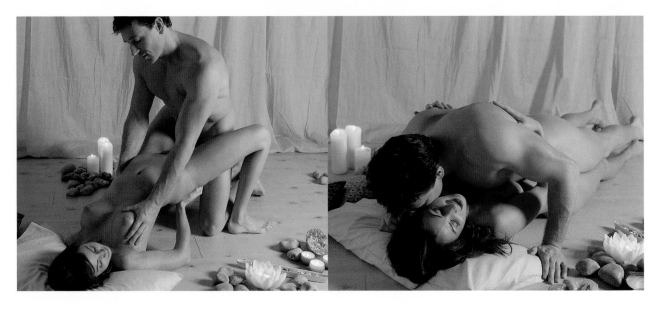

ABOVE | The flower in bloom, blossoming.

ABOVE RIGHT | The jewel case.

BELOW | Aphrodite's delight requires supple legs.

BELOW RIGHT | Dear to Cupid.

TANTRIC UNION IS A SEXUAL BOND that transcends the purely physical. Partners can forget their daily cares or status and concentrate though discipline on their being one with another person, thus achieving a higher state of ecstasy.

The positions of Tantra are based on those of the Kama Sutra. Here are a few examples translated into a more contemporary style, beginning with the supine, or lying down positions.

flower in bloom

The woman lies back, with bent knees, and spreads her legs wide, digging her heels in as close to her hips as she can. Then, placing her hands under her buttocks, she cups and lifts them with her palms, offering her yoni as a "flower in bloom". The man then enters her from between her thighs, and gently caresses her breasts. This may require some stamina and flexibility.

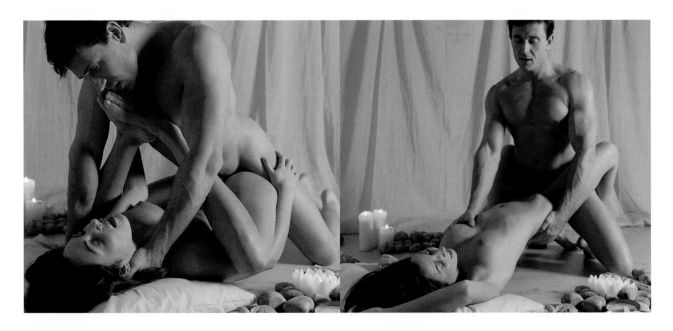

aphrodite's delight

This also requires quite a bit of flexibility from the woman. She lies back and the man clasps her feet, raising them to her breasts so that her legs form a rough circle. He then enters her, keeping her legs in place with the weight of his body, and clasps her around the neck as they make love.

dear to cupid

The woman lies back with her knees bent and the man kneels before her. He hooks her legs around his thighs and gently fondles and caresses her breasts as they make love.

the jewel case

This position is recommended for men with smaller penises. The man lies on top of the woman with his legs on top of hers, so that their legs caress each other from thighs to toes. This can either be done with the woman below the man, or side by side, in which case she should always lie to the left.

love's noose

The woman lies back as the man enters her. With her thighs pressed tightly together he encircles the woman's legs with his own. He should then squeeze and grip her thighs – very good for added clitoral stimulation.

the bud

The woman lies back and draws her legs up, clasping her knees to her breasts. This exposes her yoni (vagina) "like an opening bud" to her partner.

the mare's trick

The woman sits astride the man facing either way, and during penetration, rhythmically squeezes his penis, "milking it" with her PC muscle.

splitting the bamboo

The woman lies on her back and raises one leg over her partner's shoulder as he enters her. After a time she lowers that leg and raises the other.

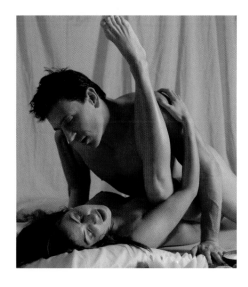

vadavaka

The art of vadavaka, or milking the man's penis, is a difficult one to be mistress of without significant practice. It can be tried in any sexual position, although some, like the mare's trick, will be easier than others where the woman is not in control.

Squeeze the PC (puboccygeus) muscle as if trying to halt the flow of urine. Pulsating in this way will heighten the pleasure of both parties. The grip may be improved by catching the glans of the lingham, or penis, behind the pubic bone, with the added advantage that it will be pushed up against the G spot here too.

ABOVE LEFT | Splitting the bamboo – this may not be comfortable for the woman for a long time, so vary the posture or move to another.

LEFT | Love's noose – this is an advanced version of the jewel case and you may find you can move between these postures quite easily.

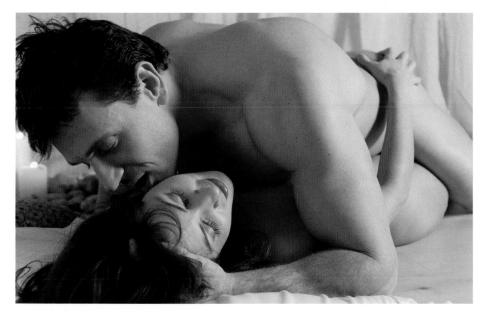

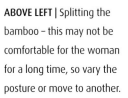

sitting tantra

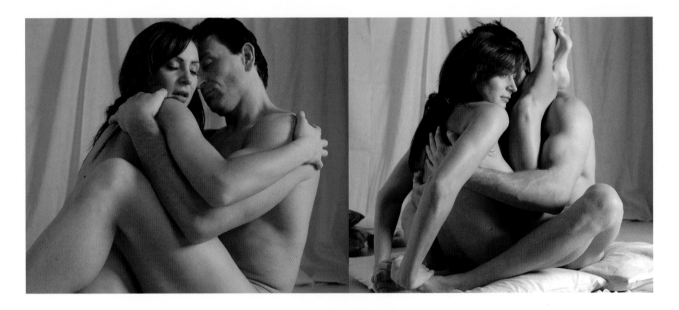

ABOVE | Feet yoke – this will be fun, once you have worked out how to do it.

ABOVE RIGHT | The lotus – it may be hard for the woman to keep her feet linked, but it isn't essential.

MANY OF THE SITTING POSITIONS are intended for long-drawn-out sex, where the couple becomes truly intertwined in mind as well as body.

the feet yoke

For this position you must both have reasonably flexible knees in order to achieve deeper penetration. The woman sits erect with one leg bent and the knee pulled in to her body, and the other leg straight out in front of her. The man does the same with opposing legs and penetrates her. If you cannot get close enough, then slip each straight leg beneath your partner's bent one, and gently pull one another closer together.

the circle

The woman sits with her left leg extended and encircles the man's waist with her right leg, laying the ankle across her left thigh. He mirrors this so that they are both entwined in a circle as they make love.

the peacock

This requires extreme female mobility! The woman sits and raises one foot to point vertically over her head, steadying it with her hand. In this position she offers up her yoni to her partner for lovemaking.

the lotus

The man and woman sit in front of each other, with his legs wrapped around the woman's waist. He then grips her ankles and locks them around the back of his neck like the link of a chain. She grips his toes or feet to steady herself as they make love.

awakening the chakras

The theory of chakras is that they are energy centres within the body that control our physical and psychological wellbeing. Kundalini energy is activated by the root chakra and allows spiritual energy to flow to the crown chakra, helping the body to achieve an ecstatic plane of consciousness.

There are seven chakras in the body. The first three, related to basic survival, are: root, associated with sexuality, pleasure and pain; belly, the central core of balance relating to sexual drive and reproduction, and solar plexus, concerned with power, intellect, will and ego. The four higher chakras relate to the mind, intellect and spirituality. The heart chakra is between the nipples, and being near the heart is associated with love, empathy and joy; the fifth, throat chakra, is associated with purity and expression; the sixth chakra, between the eyes, is often known as thethird eye and is associated with intuition, compassion and intellect; the seventh chakra is the crown chakra, found at the top of the head. It is associated with cosmic consciousness, bliss and unity.

the swing

She sits in his lap, and the man and woman hold each other's arms and take it in turns to lean backwards, until a swinging or seesaw-like rhythm is achieved. This position restricts thrusting, so is good for when the man is tired, and also for allowing both the man and woman to have an equal role in lovemaking.

striking

The woman sits astride the man, and as they make love, he strikes her chest. Suggesting that the couple hit each other may seem odd to a modern audience. In the Kama Sutra, intercourse is likened to a quarrel "on account of the contrarieties of love and its tendency to dispute." Here the striking is almost a formalized kind of role-playing, where each partner strikes the other as if in anger, increasing the blows until orgasm.

Four different types of striking are described: striking with the back of the hand; striking with fingers contracted; striking with the fist; and striking with the palm of the hand. Different sounds should be made by the recipient of the blows, such as cooing or hissing, and they should then strike back in return. Even Vatsayana was scornful of the fashion for using implements to abuse each other, calling this "painful, barbarous and base, and quite unworthy of imitation." Striking was considered another form of "external enjoyment" to be used in the throes of passion, according to the strength and the proclivities of the parties involved. Obviously, this should not be undertaken without the informed consent of one's partner.

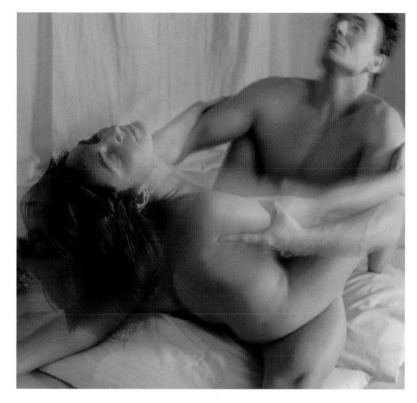

yab-yum

Yab-yum is the quintessential form of sexual union in Tantric lovemaking. It translates as "mother and father union", aligning all the energy centres (chakras) within the body, allowing kundalini energy to rise and a more spiritual level to be reached. The woman should sit on her partner's lap, facing him. Her legs should be wrapped around his waist and arms wrapped around each other. The idea is that the couple stay still and visualize, in the mind's eye, the energy rising from the root chakra to the crown, despite the temptation, of course, to move and thrust.

ABOVE | The swing can be fun once you get into the rhythm.

BELOW LEFT | Striking should be a passionate, rather than a painful, experience.

BELOW CENTRE | Yab-yum is one of the most loving poses allowing maximum contact.

BELOW | The temptation to be active can be strong.

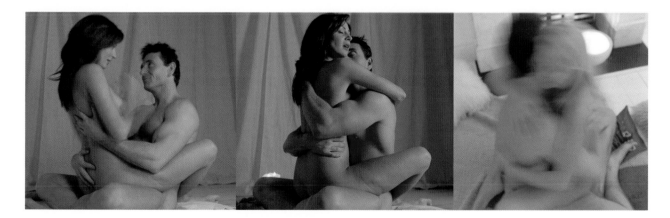

standing and rear tantra

STANDING POSITIONS were considered, by Brahmins like Vatsayana, to be a high form of congress, and they are depicted in numerous works of art. Rear entry postions were also enjoyed, taking their inspiration from the animal kingdom.

suspended

This posture requires quite a bit of strength from the man. He begins by standing with his back to a wall, but not leaning against it. The woman sits in his cradled arms with her thighs gripping his waist, feet flat against the wall and arms wrapped around his neck. As they make love she pushes back and forth against the wall.

the tripod

This requires a good sense of balance. He holds one of her knees firmly in his hand and stands, without support. As they make love she can caress and explore his body with her hands.

the dog

This is similar to the doggy position, in which the woman goes on all fours and the man enters her from behind. In Tantra, however, the woman should turn her head and gaze into her partner's eyes as they make love.

the ass

The woman stands with her legs slightly apart and bends forward, gripping her thighs with her hands, or with hands on the floor. The man then enters her from behind. Height differences can be combated by the width that she spreads her legs. For shorter men, she should spread her legs wider.

the stride

This is another one for the more adventurous and agile couple. The woman stands on her palms and feet so her body forms a triangle. From behind he lifts one of her feet to his shoulder, driving his lingham into her yoni with vigorous strokes.

the elephant

This is similar to spoons, in which the woman lies on her side facing away from the man. She offers her buttocks to him and he penetrates from behind, using his hands to gently caress the other parts of her body.

BELOW LEFT | The tripod – this is a position that could be done anywhere, but try next to the bed the first time, in case you lose your balance.

BELOW RIGHT | The ass – if the woman is not flexible enough to reach the floor, she could rest her hands on a chair.

please her yoni

It is the man's duty to please his partner and here are some suggested techniques.

manthana – churning
Grind your penis in circles once inside her, avoiding thrusting.

piditaka – pressing
Press your penis hard towards her womb and hold before withdrawing and repeating.

varahaghata – the boar's blow
Provide continuous pressure on one side of her vagina during penetration.

vrishaghata – the bull's blow
Thrust wildly in every direction while you penetrate her.

chatakavilasa – sparrow sport
Quiver your penis while it is inside her.

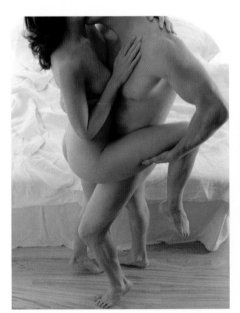

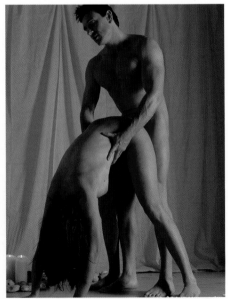

oral tantra

KNOWN AS "MOUTH CONGRESS" in the Kama Sutra, oral sex was considered a base activity practised by wanton women and eunuchs. These days it is a healthy part of most loving relationships, although some lovers are not sure how to go about it.

fellatio

There are different techniques described by Vatsayana for performing fellatio on a man. You don't have to put the whole thing in your mouth – the head is the most sensitive part.

nimitta – touching

Holding his penis with one hand, the woman shapes her mouth into an "O" and places it on the tip of her partner's penis. She moves her head in tiny circles, maintaining a light touch.

parshvatoddashta – biting to the sides

Holding the head of the penis in her hand, the woman clamps her lips lightly above the shaft, first on one side and then the other, being careful to keep her teeth hidden so as not to cause any pain.

antaha-samdansha – the inner pincers

The woman takes the whole of the head of the penis into her mouth. She then presses the shaft firmly between her lips and holds it for a few seconds before pulling away.

parimrshtaka – striking at the tip

The woman begins by flicking her tongue all over his penis, using a hard pointed tongue. Then she concentrates on the sensitive tip of the glans, striking it continually to evoke a heightened sexual sensation.

sangara – swallowed whole

This is done when the man is close to orgasm. The woman takes the whole of the penis into her mouth and sucks, working her tongue and lips until the man comes.

cunnilingus

Oral sex performed on a woman doesn't get much of a write-up in the ancient texts – it was considered just another form of kissing.

jihva-bhramanaka – the circling tongue

The man uses his nose to spread the woman's vaginal lips and then gently probes her yoni with his tongue. Then, with his nose, lips and chin, he moves in gentle circles all around her vaginal area.

chushita – sucked

The man fastens his lips to the woman's vaginal lips and nibbles at her before sucking on her clitoris. He uses varying degrees of pressure as he sucks on her clitoris until he finds one that she is comfortable with and, more importantly, one that gives her pleasure.

uchchushita – sucked up

The man cups and lifts his partner's buttocks, and uses his tongue to gently massage her navel, working down to her genitals. Once between her legs he should use his tongue to gently lap up her love juices.

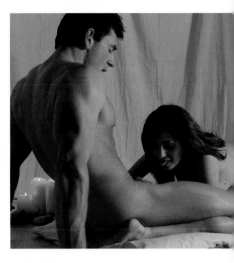

ABOVE | Striking at the tip – you don't have to put the whole penis in your mouth. The head is the most sensitive part, so concentrate here.

BELOW | Sucked up – hopefully, the tantalizing sensations will be almost unbearable by the time he reaches his destination.

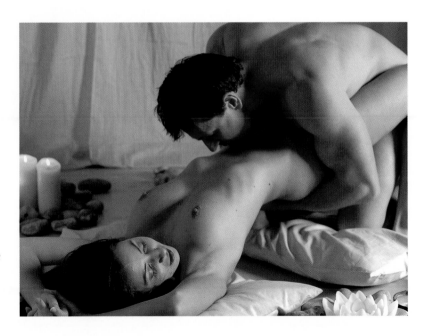

suppressing orgasm

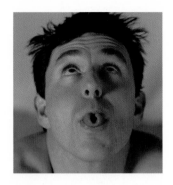

ABOVE | Controlling your breathing may help you orgasm without ejaculation.

RIGHT | Suppressing your orgasms may enable you to find an ecstatic plateau.

BELOW | Saluting one another acknowledges the other's body as the bridge to the spiritual world.

ACHIEVING ORGASM is often seen as the *sine qua non* of modern sex. Without that emphasis, lovemaking can become more relaxed and less goal-orientated. So sex without orgasm can be an activity in itself. Each partner tries not to reach orgasm for as long as possible.

The Tantric skill of maithuna is a technique for controlling response, designed to help intensify orgasm and also to help men to delay their orgasm to keep in harmony with their partner's sexual tempo. The technique is designed to help the flow of sexual energy and to ensure men feel energized after sex as opposed to exhausted.

● When you feel like you are about to come, breathe deeply. Many people hold their breath, as if forcing the orgasm to come out. By keeping the breathing regular the orgasm will become more intense as you flow with and not against it.

● Keep the tip of your tongue on the roof of your mouth or roll it into a "straw" to breathe through. This can help to circulate the energy and help men to withhold their orgasm.

● When you begin to orgasm, imagine the energy is flowing away from your genitals and up your spine. Do not contort yourself to try and help this physically. This is purely a visualization to

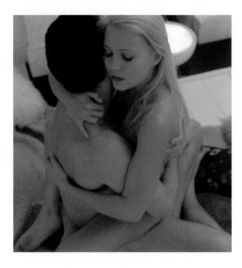

prolong orgasm. The more control a man has over his own sexual responses, the more he will be able to offer his partner.

saluting one another

At the culmination of your time together, you should sit before each other and salute each other, saying words such as, "You are a god/goddess." This acknowledges the other's body and gives praise for awakening each other's senses, and thanks for helping each other in the unity of spiritual Tantric lovemaking.

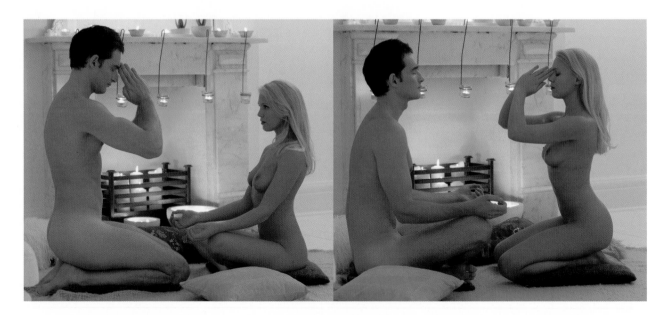

tantric energy orgasms

ENERGY ORGASMS CLEANSE THE BODY of repression, emotional pain and sexual blocks and barricades. It is a Tantric masturbation technique that requires deep concentration, visualization and lots of practice. Energy orgasms can vary in strength – extra time put into building energy generally leads to a more powerful orgasm. It is for men and women, and is said to be very different from an ordinary orgasm and may or may not feel sexual.

move like a butterfly

Begin by lying on a flat hard surface and bend your knees up. Start to take a few deeper breaths, empty your mind and release the tension in your mind and body. As you inhale, arch your lower back to rock your pelvis, and as you exhale, squeeze your PC (puboccygeus) muscle. (These are the muscles that stop the flow of urine when you pee.) By squeezing these muscles you are stimulating the G spot and clitoris or penis and testicles, and at the same time you are helping to pump energy throughout your body. Let your breathing and contractions be erotic and as you repeat the circular breathing technique, fan your legs open as you inhale and close as you exhale, like butterfly wings, to help to keep the energy flowing and maintain your rhythm.

Your energy will follow your thought processes, so visualize drawing energy in from the atmosphere and into the perineum area, between your genitals and anus. Build strong fires of energy in the sex centres of the first and second chakras and circulate this energy back and forth. Once the energy feels powerful and strong, move it up and continue circulating it from the genital area to the belly area, the first and second chakras. Again, once you feel that the energy is strong, let it flow from the belly to the heart, the fourth chakra, via the solar plexus, the third. Then move the circulating energy on from the heart to the fifth, throat, chakra. You may find it helpful to consciously make sounds, opening the throat and allowing energy to then circulate upwards from the throat to the third eye, circulating between the fifth and sixth chakras.

Finally, visualize the energy flowing between the third eye and the top of the head, the seventh, crown, chakra. Now you should start to feel the energy shoot from the top of your head and a full body orgasm will hopefully begin stirring. Follow the flow of the orgasm. Your breathing patterns may change and with practice you will learn to ride the waves of your orgasm and allow them to keep it going for longer and longer periods of time.

Don't worry if you don't reach orgasm first time round. This is a technique that requires a lot of practice. The breathing exercises alone will reap their own benefits by cleansing your mind of mental blocks and hurtful memories, clearing the path for more positive orgasmic experiences.

BELOW | It may be helpful to do some further research on the chakras so that you will know what you are trying to visualize. Each chakra is distinguished by a colour and a frequency of vibration which will become familiar to you as you practise.

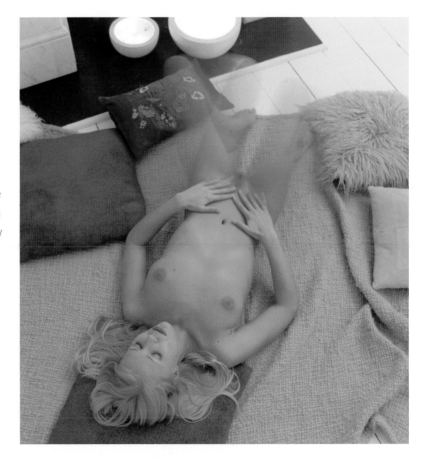

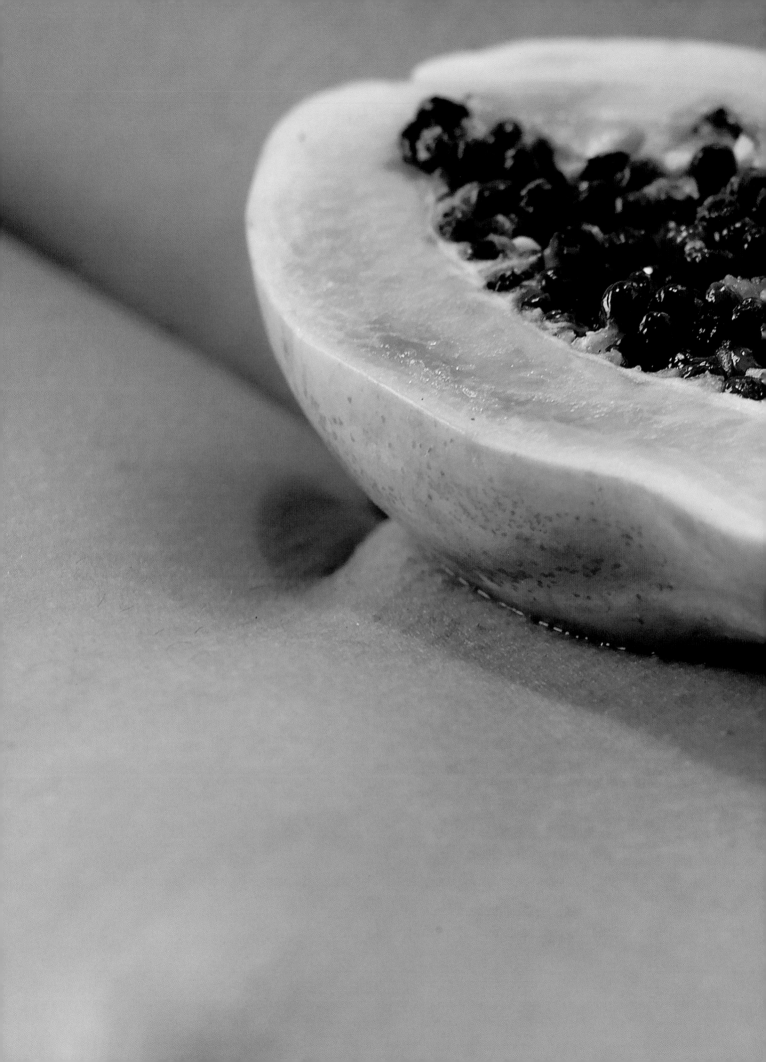

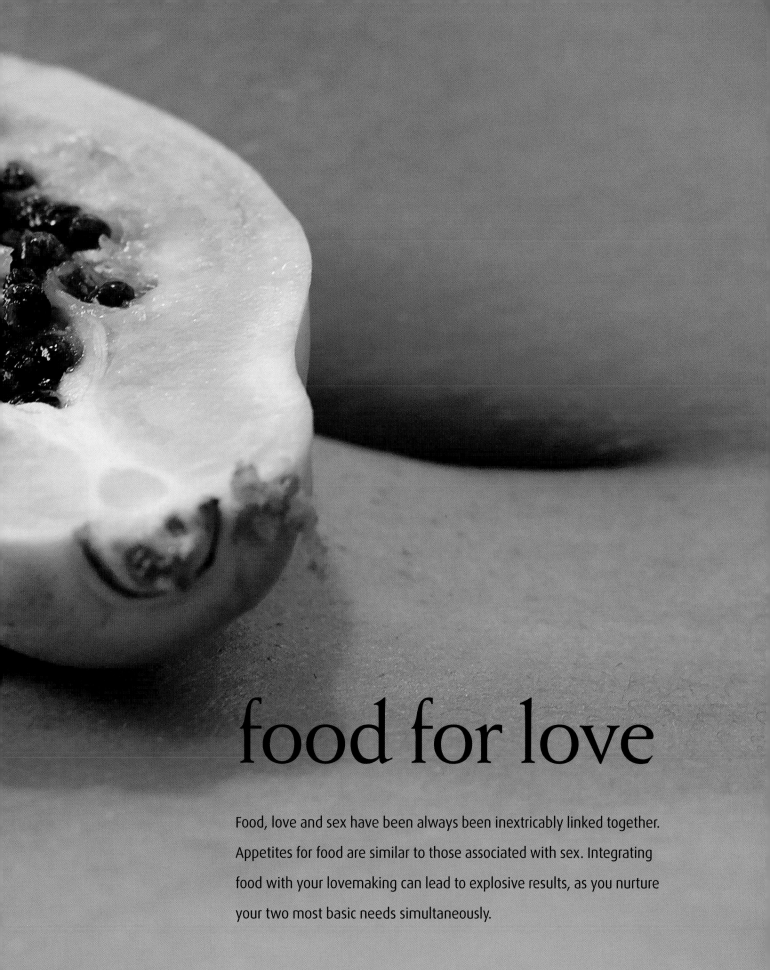

food for love

Food, love and sex have been always been inextricably linked together.
Appetites for food are similar to those associated with sex. Integrating
food with your lovemaking can lead to explosive results, as you nurture
your two most basic needs simultaneously.

food and sex

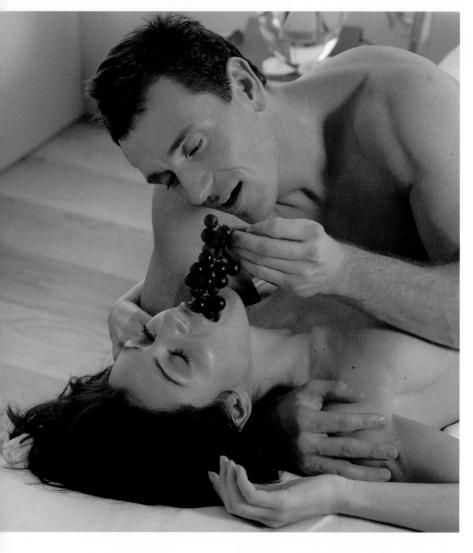

ABOVE | Food and sex are inextricably linked and sharing food with your partner is one of the most intimate things you can do.

WHERE WOULD ROMANCE BE without the element of food? We even use foodie words to describe people we are attracted to: she's a peach, or he's really tasty, scrumptious or delicious. Honey, sugar and my sweet are terms of endearment. The reason that food has always played a part in the rituals of courtship is that both eating and sex are two of our strongest instincts and a combination of both can prove irresistible. Food, like sex, is another way of stimulating the senses. The flavour and taste, the texture and touch, the visual appearance, the aromas and even sound of food cooking, all play a part in its sensual appeal.

Part of the excitement of courtship is finding out about each other. You can tell so much about the person you are with from the food they buy, the method in which they cook and present it, what they choose from the menu in a restaurant and how they eat it. People with hearty appetites who really enjoy their food often have a healthy appetite for sex as well.

We use our mouths for many different things – talking, kissing, sucking, smiling, laughing, as well as eating – so watching your partner slide the flesh of an oyster into their mouth and imagining the salty, silken texture slipping down their throat can be very arousing. Eating draws attention to the mouth. The tongue, the lips and genitals all have the same neural receptors, called Kraus's end bulbs, which make them supersensitive to stimulation. This is why kissing is such an important part of the prelude to lovemaking.

a lovers' menu

Of course, we eat with our eyes as well as our mouths. The shape of certain foods can be very erotic and can conjure up all manner of suggestive images; a downy peach looks like a voluptuous bottom, oysters and figs are reminiscent of a woman's vulva, and bananas, celery and asparagus are phallic. Some foods just look irresistible – think of sashimi or chocolate cake.

In fact all the senses come into play. The pervasive aroma of truffles is astonishingly sensuous, while the sweet scent of strawberries or mangoes makes the mouth water. Texture is as important as flavour and intrinsically sexy foods include: caviar that just bursts on the tongue; anything that you eat with your fingers from a chicken drumstick to edamame (soya beans); most shellfish from scallops to crayfish, although not anything you have to remove with a pin. The sound of food sizzling stirs the appetites. There is something strangely erotic about the crunch when your lover bites into an apple.

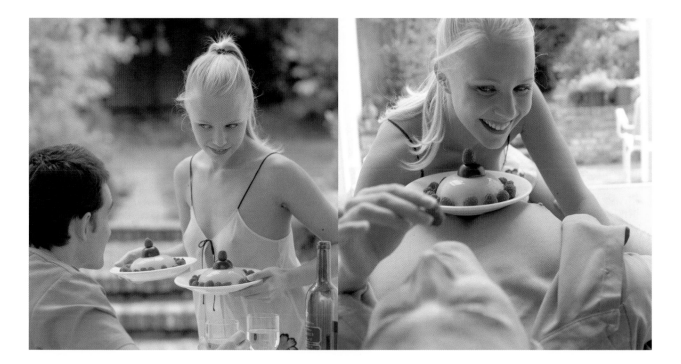

Don't forget that what you drink matters, too. Champagne is a turn-on for most people, cocktails are glamorous and even a mug of creamy hot chocolate after a brisk walk on a windy day can stir the senses. The light sparkling on beautiful crystal glasses adds to the sensuous pleasure of good wine, while many men find the sight of their partners drinking "designer" beer straight from the bottle very arousing. Drinking tequila the traditional way is sexy and fun: place a little salt on the back of your hand between your index finger and thumb and hold a wedge of lime in the same hand, then lick the salt, down a shot of tequila in one and then suck the lime.

saucy snacks

Sex shops sell a range of naughty nibbles, including chocolate body paint and penis-, bottom- and breast-shaped chocolates, combining everybody's favourite aphrodisiac with an element of fun. You can even buy edible underwear.

With a little imagination, you can create your own suggestive dishes. How about setting pink blancmange in shallow, 15cm/6in dishes and, when they're turned out, topping with them with glacé (candied) cherry nipples? Then just try serving them without a sly smile.

sexy cocktails

Why not dress up for cocktail hour? One of you can be the bartender, and the other the Hollywood starlet. Each of these recipes will make one cocktail.

- **slippery nipple** – Stir 1 measure Bailey's Irish Cream with ice. Strain into a cocktail glass and float 1 tsp Sambuca on top.
- **sex on the beach** – Pour 2 measures vodka, 1 measure peach brandy, 2 measures cranberry juice and 1 measure mixed orange and pineapple juice into a cocktail shaker over ice. Shake vigorously, then strain into a tall glass and decorate with a slice of orange.
- **slow comfortable screw up against the wall** – Fill a highball glass with ice cubes, then pour in 2 measures sloe gin and top up with fresh orange juice. Float 1 tsp Galliano on top.
- **bosom caresser** – Dash a little Cointreau over ice in a jug, pour in 1 measure brandy and 1 measure Madeira. Stir and strain into a glass.

ABOVE | Provocative, if not subtle: create your own range of suggestive snacks and find imaginative ways of serving and eating them.

BELOW | Why not try a slow comfortable screw up against the wall – then you'll really need a drink.

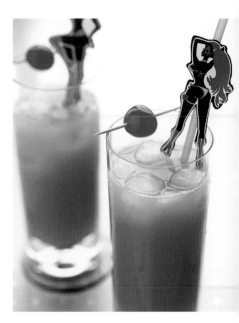

aphrodisiacs

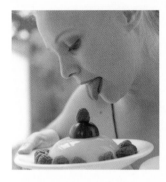

ABOVE | Food can be about more than nutrition.

RIGHT | Any Italian will tell you that spaghetti is one of the sexiest foods around, even if one of the messiest.

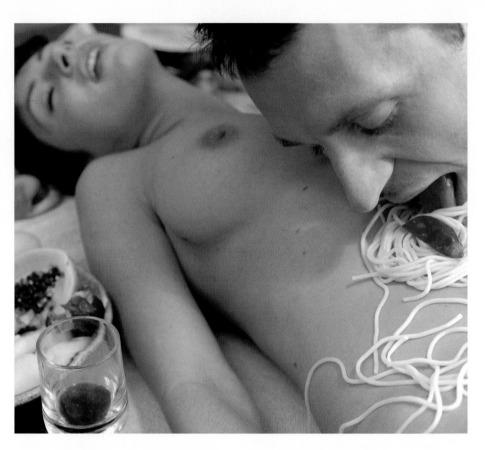

SINCE TIME IMMEMORIAL, men and women have been obsessive in their search for the ultimate aphrodisiac to help flagging libidos, improve their sexual performance and generally enhance the act of lovemaking.

Ayurvedic medicine, which originated in ancient India, so valued the importance of sex that a whole branch of medicine was dedicated to it called "Vajikarana", and there is a wide spectrum of preparations in use around the world that use animals and insects to enhance sexual performance. The Romans ate the penises, wombs and testes of animals such as monkeys, pigs, cockerels and goats, and lizards used to be pulverized and the powder taken with sweet white wine by the Arabs and southern Europeans. The Chinese today often use the genitals of animals and insects to increase the strength of reproductive organs, believing that ingesting

substances with sexual properties will impart those properties to the person consuming them. Snake blood is still consumed in east Asian countries and the gallstones of animals are used in Asian countries alongside ginseng and royal jelly.

chocoholic

Of course, it's debatable whether any aphrodisiacs actually work – there's certainly very little scientific evidence – but most people would draw the line at powdered reptiles and foul-tasting herbs. Fortunately, there is an extensive range of far more palatable options.

On the Richter scale of aphrodisiacs, chocolate is up there among the top three, alongside champagne and oysters. People are passionate about it. The Aztecs brewed cocoa like coffee, and Aztec leader Montezuma is alleged to have drunk up to 50 cups a day so that he could keep going with his harem of 600 women. It may have gained its reputation because the Aztecs believed the cacao pod was a symbol of the human heart. The notorious Marquis de Sade is said to have demanded chocolate cake while imprisoned. Chocolate lovers will gladly eat it before, during and after sex and some even choose it instead of sex. But what is it about chocolate that is so special? It's questionable that it can really affect sexual performance, but it does possess certain stimulating properties. As you swallow it, a chemical called phenylethylamine and the feel-good neurotransmitter serotonin are released in your brain, spreading a feeling of tranquillity. Then, the theobromine in chocolate kicks in to create the high feeling that you have when you are in love. Chocolate also contains other stimulants, such as caffeine, which excite the central nervous system, but all these properties exist in such tiny amounts that you would have to consume vast quantities for it to have any real sexual effect. What is certain is that chocolate contains sugar, which provides energy, and that, combined with its pleasurable texture and flavour, may explain why so many people find it so addictive. For many women, the fact that it is a "forbidden food" is also exciting.

foods for sex

Champagne, of course, like any alcoholic drink, reduces inhibitions, but too much will cause a downturn in your sex life. Oysters, on the other hand, have a long-standing reputation for stimulating the libido. This is undoubtedly much to do with their appearance and texture, but, interestingly, they are extremely rich in zinc, "the sex mineral" essential for the production of healthy sperm and fertility. Scallops also contain high levels of zinc and have a reputation for increasing the sex drive in women. In fact, aphrodisiac qualities have been ascribed to seafood of various sorts, including lobsters and caviar, while Chinese medicine recommends mussels and shrimps for increasing the libido.

Many foods, such as asparagus, morel mushrooms, figs and avocados, have been thought to possess such properties simply as a result of their appearance. Others, such as salmon and pigeon, seem to have been designated as aphrodisiacs because of the living creature's courtship rituals. The reasons for the reputation of still further foods are even more mysterious. The Romans swore by bread, which may have been because eating a lot of it tends to make you want to lie down. However, eating a lot of it also promotes flatulence, which is distinctly unsexy. When tomatoes were first imported into Europe, the French called them love apples for their heart-like shape. Nevertheless, tomatoes are high in lycopene, which is essential for prostate health. The Chinese recommend ginger and this too has a grain of validity in that it promotes healthy circulation, especially to the genitals.

So do aphrodisiacs really work? It seems unlikely, but their placebo effect can work wonders and, as we all know, the most powerful aphrodisiac that exists is the imagination.

BELOW | In different cultures and throughout history, a range of foods have been thought to raise the libido. Certainly some foods have an erotic sensuousness and sharing them with your lover can be very arousing.

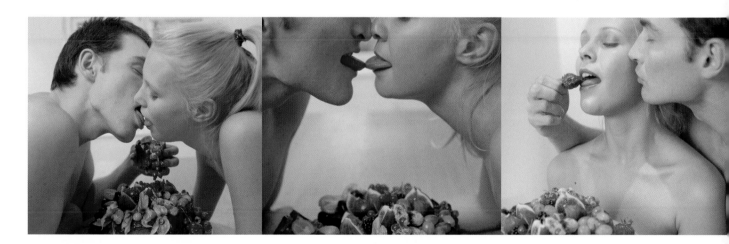

foodplay

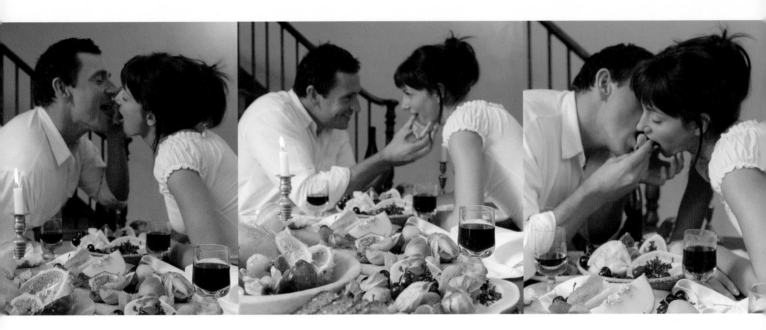

ABOVE | Choose the tastiest morsels and most succulent treats and feed them to your partner with your fingers or your lips.

OPPOSITE | A truly seductive meal can easily turn out to be more than metaphorical foreplay and you may not be able to wait to clear the table.

WHEN PLANNING A PASSIONATE evening with your partner, think of your meal as part of the foreplay to your lovemaking. Never underestimate the importance of food and wine in the enjoyment of a romantic evening. Teasing each other across a candlelit table can be so tantalizing. The cardinal rules for eating before sex are never to eat too much and never to select food that is too heavy. No one wants to make love on a full stomach – their own or someone else's.

Sharing your food and feeding each other is a potent form of foreplay. Having a romantic meal in the privacy of your own home is a wonderful opportunity for you to be outrageous flirts and to act out your seductive desires. You both know what's coming, but so much of the enjoyment is in the getting there.

Set the scene beforehand. Make the table look enticing with a lovely cloth, some flowers and candles, but don't use your best china as it may get swept to the floor in the heat of the moment.

Because no one else is there, you can act out your romantic fantasies and pull out all the seductive stops. Remember all those scenes in movies which you have always wanted to try out?

Well, now here's your chance. Think Jennifer Beals in *Flashdance* or Mickey Rourke and Kim Basinger in *9½ Weeks*, rather than Meg Ryan in *When Harry Met Sally*. It's also a perfect opportunity to tell each other things that you don't necessarily say over the breakfast cereal. In this romantic setting you remind one another just how much you still desire each other. Don't forget the music. It should be romantic, sexy and not too loud, something that is meaningful to both of you.

gourmet sex

The whole process of eating can be incorporated into the art of seduction. Start your sensuous feast with pre-dinner drinks and little canapés as light as butterfly kisses. Next, the appetizer should be a tantalizing treat, promising much more and seducing you with its textures and flavours. The main course is the climax of the meal, satisfying but not satiating your appetite, while dessert is a pause for refreshment.

Playing with the stem of your glass, running your fingertips around the rim and stroking the stem has its own connotations. Locking eyes with your lover over your glass of wine, caressing his or her hand across the table, making soft moans and sighs of pleasure as you enjoy an asparagus tip dripping with butter, even the way you butter your roll, can all create a tremendous sexual tension between the two of you. As the meal progresses and the wine diminishes, you can become bolder, eating off each other's plates or kissing the traces of food from each other's lips. End this wonderful meal by feeding each other delicious morsels of fresh fruit, passing them from mouth to mouth and allowing the juices to flow. Lots of action can take place under the table as well as on top. Kick off your shoes and caress each other's feet and legs.

finger foods

There is always something especially sexy about eating with your fingers, perhaps because we were always told not to do it when we were children. The only places where it is acceptable are fast food outlets, which must be among the least seductive locations on the planet.

If you're not in the mood for a three-course meal, then prepare a mini-banquet of succulent snacks that you can eat with your fingers – or better still, feed each other with your fingers. In fact, why not keep a ready supply of enticing nibbles in the refrigerator for just such occasions?

Include your partner's favourite rude food as well as your own. For the purposes of erotic eating, you can interpret the words "finger food" very loosely. Fruit is a perfect choice. Try wedges of watermelon or slices of mango and then lick the juices that have run over your partner's hands or chin. Bite into a strawberry or lychee and then offer your mouth to your partner.

weekend break

At the other end of the day, treating yourselves to a leisurely breakfast in bed at the weekend is a deliciously indulgent experience. It needs a little advanced planning, otherwise by the time it is ready, the mood will have been lost. The night before, prepare a tray with cups, saucers and plates, knives, spoons, marmalade or jam and, perhaps, a single flower in a small vase. Set the coffee maker ready to switch on and make sure that you have some croissants or rolls to pop into the oven in the morning. Avoid bowls of cereal, both messy and unromantic, and toast, which produces uncomfortable crumbs.

Don't take the newspapers back to bed with you and forget morning television, although some quiet background music could be atmospheric. That way, when you have finished eating, you'll have to think of something else to do.

fruity

Of all the food groups, it is fruit that is most closely associated with sensual pleasure. Grapes, the fleshy fruit, are associated with the ancient gods Dionysus, Priapus and Bacchus, the true connoisseurs of sex and pleasure. Across North Africa and the Middle East, dates are believed to increase erotic potency in men and desire in women. Coconuts are believed in India to increase the quality and quantity of semen. Strawberries and raspberries invite you to feed your lover, piece by piece. But it is fleshy fruits such as papaya, mango, peaches and apricots which spill over into true, and outrageously sticky, sensuality.

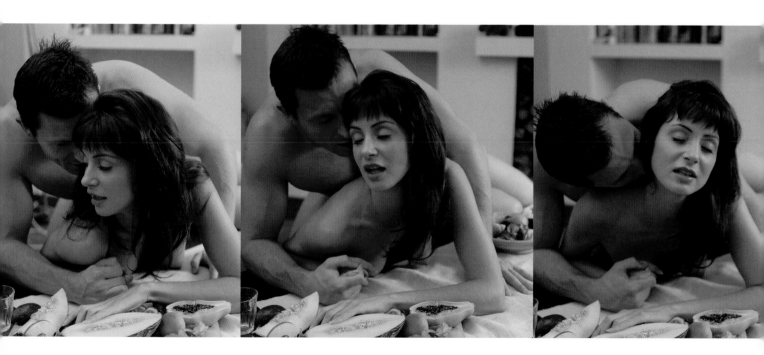

cooking with your lover

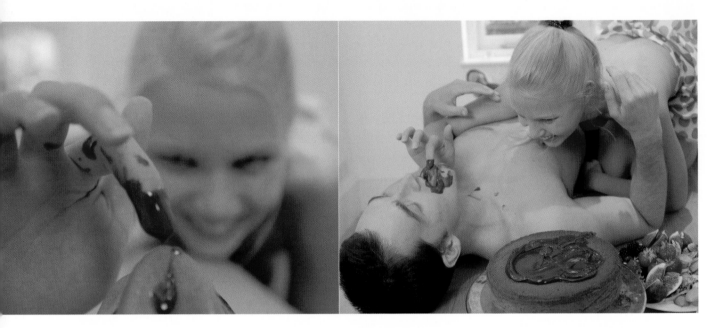

ABOVE | Nothing quite comes close to the taste and texture of molten chocolate.

ABOVE RIGHT | Making a cake to share with your partner can be just as much fun as eating it afterwards.

BELOW | Once the main course is cooking in the oven and the dessert is prepared, it's time to turn up the heat.

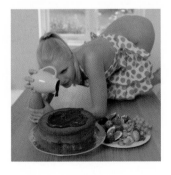

COOKING TOGETHER can bring an extra romantic dimension and sense of intimacy to the whole process of eating. Lots of people don't really enjoy the nitty gritty of food preparation, but when it's done together, you can make it much more fun. Put on some music, open a bottle of wine and get your ingredients together.

Choosing the ingredients that suit your mood at the time adds to the joy of sharing the cooking experience. It's fun to shop together, especially at an outdoor market, where you can handle the produce and ponder over which particular item you think is best. You can linger over plump, bright red tomatoes and let yourselves be seduced by the smell of ripe cantaloupe melons or fresh juicy mangoes.

If you are adventurous, it's a great turn-on to try to cook something totally different. Leave plenty of time for the preparation and have an adventure in the kitchen while you are chopping, slicing and stirring.

This is a wonderful opportunity for some serious love play as well, as you add a pinch of seduction to the list of ingredients. While the chocolate cake is rising in the oven you could be stripping down to your sexy underwear or negligee. For the truly adventurous, why not strip off totally and cook wearing nothing more than an apron? Take Isabel Allende's advice in her book *Aphrodite*: "Everything cooked for a lover is sensual, but it is even more so if both take part in the preparation and seize the opportunity to naughtily shed a garment or two as the onions are peeled or leaves stripped from the artichokes."

man about the house

Recent research has revealed that women are turned on by men who cook and you have only to think of the devoted female following of the many male celebrity chefs on television to see a clear manifestation of this. Women undoubtedly have a more emotional attitude towards food than men, so when a man is wielding a whisk or chopping a chilli, he is not just entering traditional female physical territory, but also her psychological home ground, which can be very alluring.

Another study by the Smell and Taste Treatment and Research Center in Chicago may provide an additional incentive to any men reluctant to enter the kitchen until the meal is on the table. The aroma of different foods as they cook has, apparently, a profound effect on the libido and, in particular, the smell of meat cooking significantly increases the flow of blood to the penis. This fact could make basting the Sunday roast a whole lot more fun.

feasting the senses

Cooking shouldn't be a chore, but it can often seem to be, particularly when it's a routine responsibility. Cooking with your partner can change this, especially if you tackle the task with a new attitude, actively relishing the textures, colours, smells and flavours of your ingredients. Preparing food can be as sensuous as eating it, especially when you are sharing the experience. Try out some new recipes, adding your own special touches, inhaling the aromas and tasting as you go. Does the chocolate mousse need more

orange juice? Dip in your finger and hold it out for your partner to decide. By the time they've finished licking it clean, they will probably have forgotten the question. Waft a spoonful of your newly created sauce beneath their nose, but tantalizingly deny them a taste until they have guessed at least three of the spices that flavour it.

Enjoy sharing the sensations of cooking and encourage each other to be daring in the kitchen. If you've never attempted to toss a pancake, try it and see who can catch it. Ice a cake together – literally, if you like, squeezing your partner's hands and the icing bag at the same time. Messy, but fun. Get out the food colouring and see who can create the most outrageous masterpiece with the mashed potatoes. Food is one of our most basic needs, and we all know how important it is to have a balanced diet, but you can still have a lot of fun together while you are preparing it.

BELOW | Experimenting together and tasting the fruits of each other's labours makes cooking together fun.

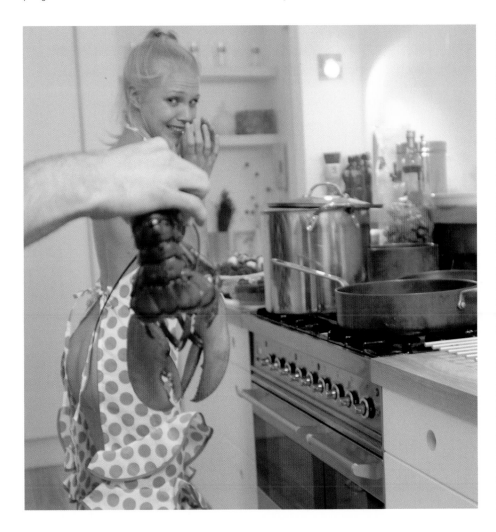

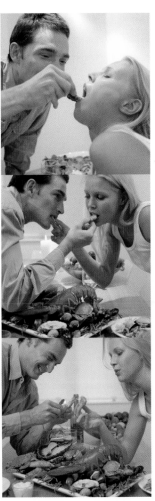

food without plates

THE MOST EROTIC WAY to share food with a lover is when you are both totally naked, so that you can eat from each other's bodies. It's a mutual experience. Where one enjoys the sensation of having food eaten from their body, the other enjoys the application and the subsequent pleasure of eating off their lover's body without using their hands.

What food you use is a question of personal taste. Many people enjoy the cool, silky sensation of cream or yogurt being drizzled over their body before being slowly licked off. Honey is another favourite, especially when massaged into the breasts before being nuzzled off. Smooth peanut butter can be warmed and smoothed over the penis (avoiding the urethral opening). Take your time slowly to suck it and lick it off. If you have a sweet tooth, you may prefer to use vanilla ice cream or strawberry jam. (These might prompt a much more dramatic response, as neurological research has shown that the smells of these two substances increase penile blood flow by anything up to 40 per cent.) Be creative when laying the food across the skin. Use a mixture of flavours, textures, aromas, tastes and temperatures. Cover your lover's naked body with slices of your favourite fruit or vegetables or make patterns with melted chocolate and eat them off.

If you really want to go for it and have a full body banquet, one of you can be the main course and the other the dessert. Don't eat very much the day before, make sure you have everything within easy reach and leave yourselves plenty of time. In between courses, you can have a long leisurely bath together, to be relaxed and receptive for the next course. Be especially mindful when you come to the more sensitive, delicate regions of the body such as the eyes, the vagina and the penis. Avoid any acidic, astringent irritants, such as vinegar, pickles or lemon juice, and particularly never use any form of chilli where it may sting.

BELOW | Asparagus is an age-old sexual remedy for men and there is nutritional evidence that it can assist in regulating hormonal balance. Mushrooms are a good source of the vitamin B complex, while truffles smell fantastic.

BELOW RIGHT AND OPPOSITE | Turn your partner into a banqueting table and feast off their bare body before offering your own for dessert.

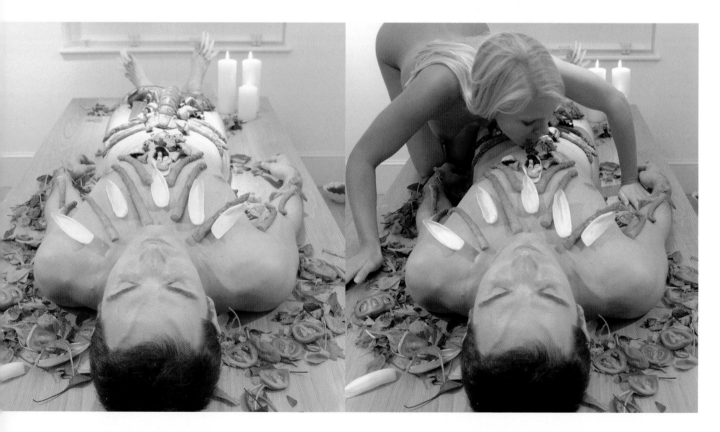

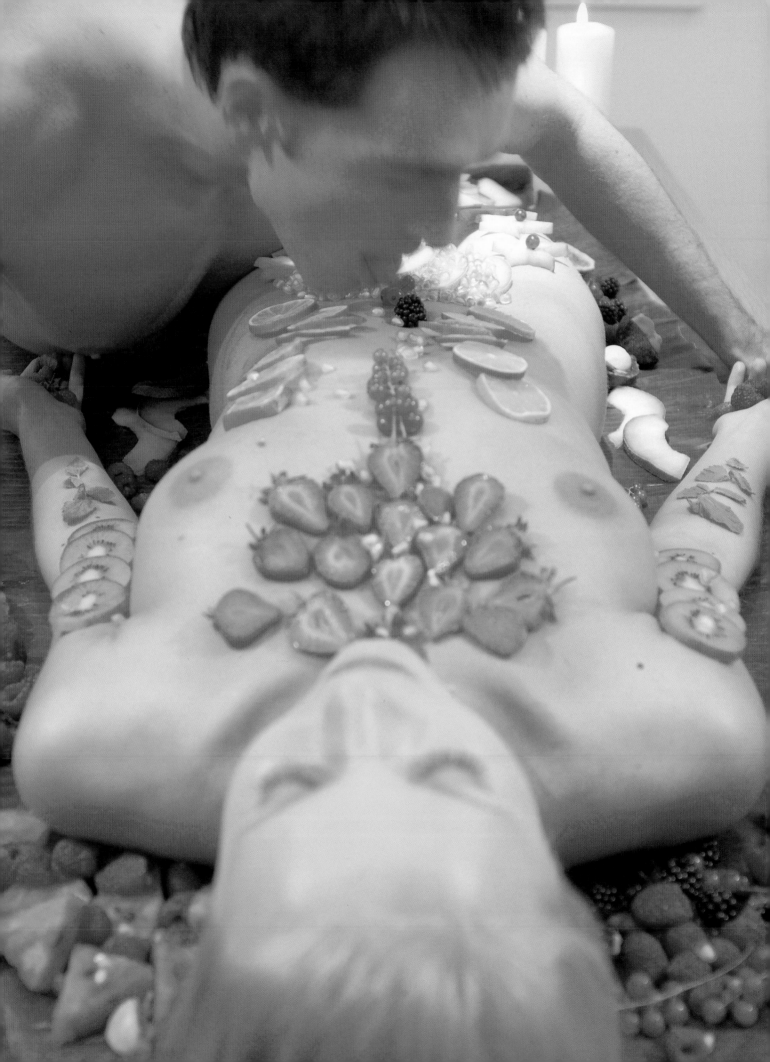

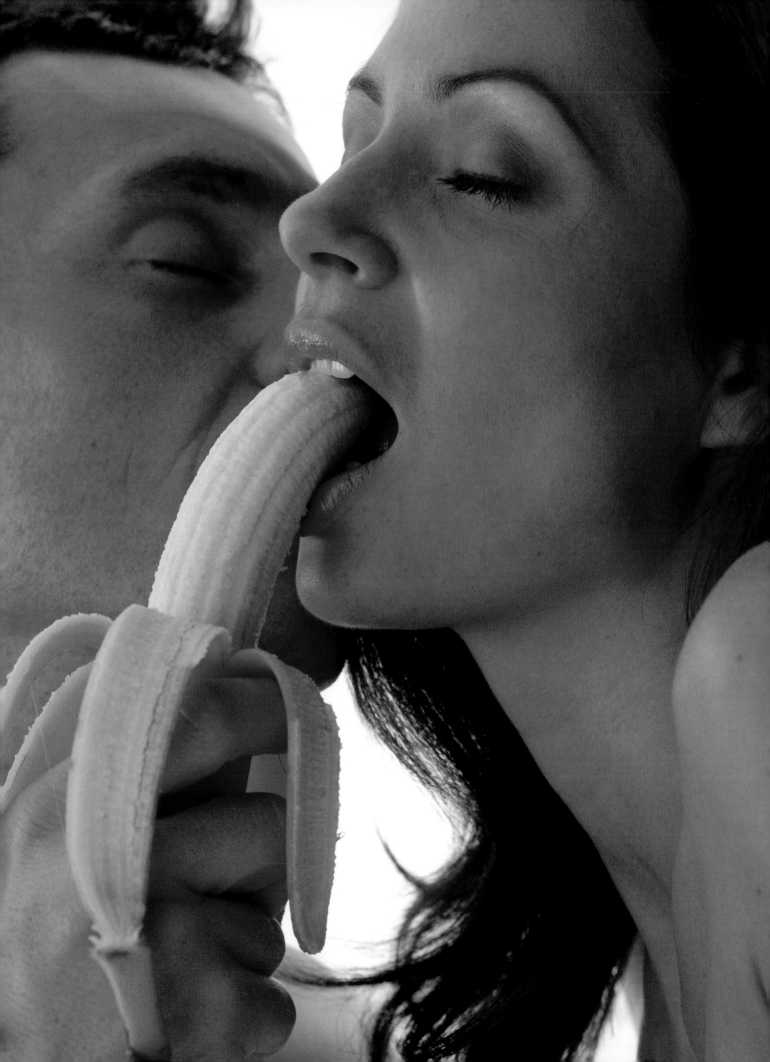

good food, good sex

FOOD ISN'T JUST FOR FUN AND SEX – it helps your body to stay on top of things. Eating well is essential to good sexual health and function. There are many, many reasons for loss of libido and impaired sexual function, but often one of the primary reasons is the balance of our sex hormones. However, this balance is also linked to our metabolic hormones, and these rely on a constant supply of certain nutrients that we provide through our diet.

minerals

Important dietary minerals include iron, zinc, magnesium, calcium, iodine, selenium, chromium, arginine, co-enzyme Q10 and essential fatty acids (EFAs). There are many food sources that are rich in these minerals. For example, chicken and red meat are rich in iron, which is needed for haemoglobin production in blood, essential for arousal, erection and lubrication. Nuts, brown rice, eggs and cheese all contain zinc, from which the sperm's tail is formed, so helping with fertility and sexual performance. Shellfish, dried fruit and dairy produce all contain calcium, crucial for bone growth and cardiovascular health and an essential ingredient for arousal, as it plays a part in sending messages to the nerves, enabling the sensation of touch. It is also needed for the contractions of muscle during male and female orgasm.

vitamins

In helping to maintain physical and sexual health, vitamins such as vitamin A, vitamin B complex (including B_1, B_2, B_3, B_5, B_6, B_{12} and choline), vitamin C and vitamin E all have their own roles.

Spinach, watercress, dairy produce and oily fish all contain vitamin A, which is vital for healthy eyes and strong bones and teeth. It is also an antioxidant required for cardiovascular health. Pulses, nuts, avocados and meat contain vitamin B complex such as B_3, which helps the circulation, allowing more blood to specific areas, such as the penis during erection; B_6, which plays an important role in regulating sex hormone function such as testosterone in men; and choline, which helps with transmission of nerve impulses necessary for boosting libido and energy during sex. Vitamin C helps to boost sex drive and strengthen male and female sex organs and can be found in food such as potatoes, ginger, beetroot (beet), citrus fruit and sprouted beans. Vitamin E is essential for healthy skin and its protective nature makes it vital for sexual health and vitality. It can be found in avocados, spinach, wheatgerm and all leafy green vegetables.

A good basic principle is to always have a balanced diet and to eat small portions regularly. Sex on a very full stomach is never a good idea.

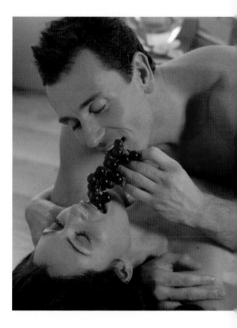

ABOVE AND OPPOSITE | it's the way that you eat it that counts.

BELOW | There are certain elements which are crucial to keep body and soul together, and without which a healthy sex life would be impossible. Nutritionally speaking, fruit and seafood are some of the richest foods.

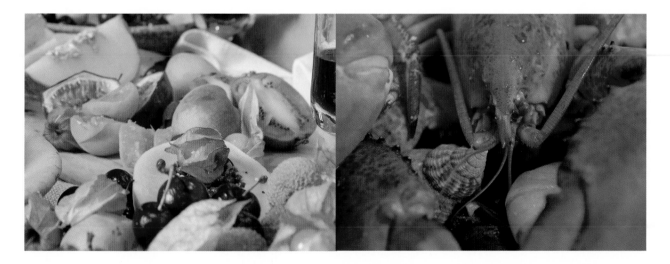

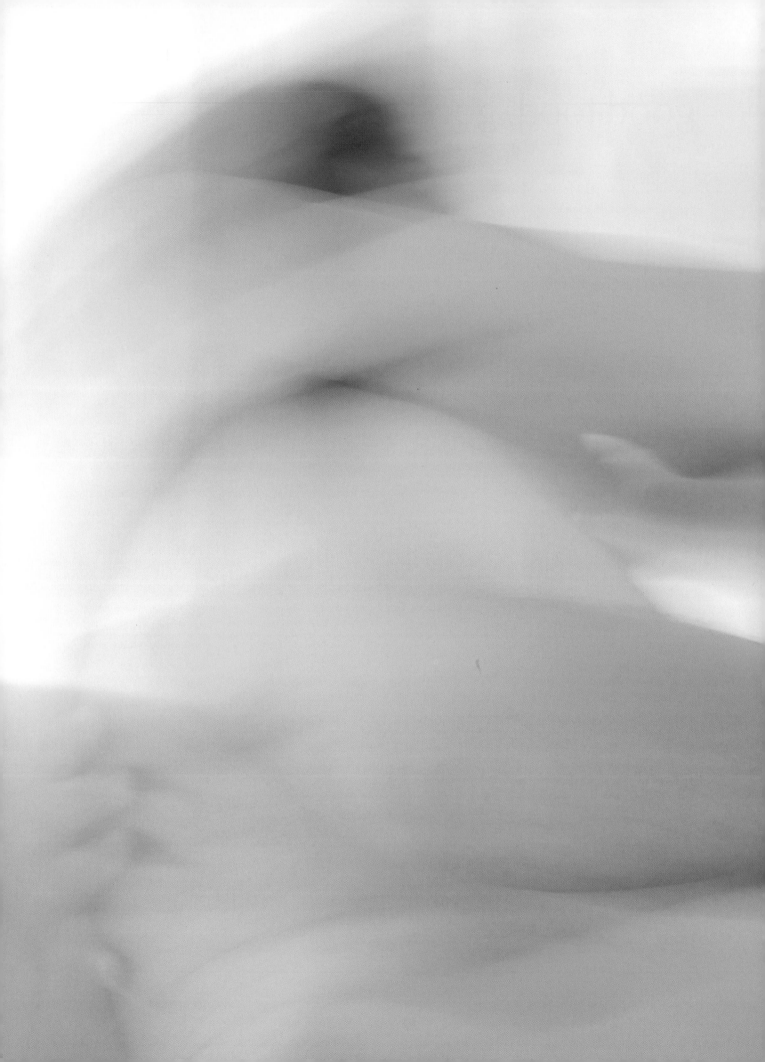

sexual health

Good sex is usually invigorating and energetic and therefore needs to be backed up by a fit body. Eating the right food and taking exercise can help people cope with life's challenges, maintaining energy and vitality in their sex lives. Taking responsibility for contraception and practising safer sex is also important to staying healthy.

bedroom workout

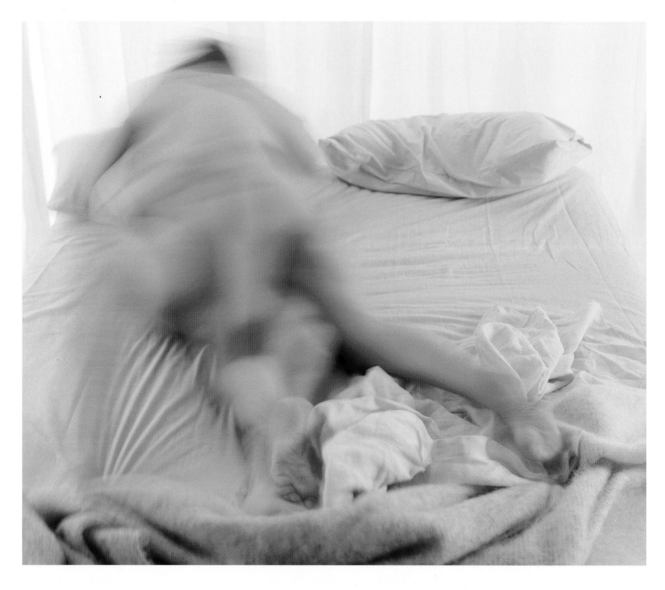

ABOVE | Lovemaking is a workout in itself, but it will be all the more pleasurable – and frequent – if you exercise to keep yourself fit and supple.

GOOD HEALTH MEANS GOOD SEX. Regular exercise promotes energy and stamina. If you are feeling good about yourself and your body, then you can feel good about your sex life, whatever age you happen to be.

There appears to be a direct relationship between being a couch potato and a lack of sexual potency. Research in the USA on a group of middle-aged men who led sedentary lives found that just one hour of exercise three times a week greatly improved their sexual function in terms of frequency, orgasm and satisfaction. Similarly, a

study of women in their forties who exercised regularly revealed that they had more frequent and enjoyable sex than women of the same age who did not exercise.

Sex is, of course, a form of exercise in itself, needing cardiovascular and muscle fitness, so exercise is important for that reason alone. And one of the many benefits of sex is that it is actually a fantastic workout that helps to keep you fit. The average person's heartbeat is around 70 beats per minute, and during lovemaking this can increase to up to 150 beats per minute, about the same as an athlete's heart rate during maximum effort. Really vigorous sex is the equivalent of 15–20 minutes on the running machine, and burns around 200 calories, which is why many people feel hungry after sex. The contractions of your pelvic and other muscles during sex also help to strengthen and tone these muscles.

fitness regime

In order to maintain an active sex life as we age and slow down, it is necessary to supplement our carnal workout with other fitness regimes. Vigorous exercise, such as running or swimming, for half an hour or more, three times a week, helps to keep everyone mentally and physically fitter. Your level of mobility and state of health will dictate the sort of activities that you should do. Whether it is a brisk walk or cycle, or a trip to the gym to use equipment such as the treadmill or rowing machine, all will help to increase your own personal fitness level.

A regular fitness regime not only helps to keep your muscular and cardiac systems healthy but also has many other benefits – helping to lower stress and blood cholesterol levels and reducing the risk of heart disease, high blood pressure, strokes and diabetes. It also increases your muscle and bone strength and your flexibility. These benefits not only help you keep sexually active for longer, but also help you to practise positions that may previously have been too difficult for you to try.

It is never too late to start exercising, although it is better to start a regime before you actually experience problems. People can begin exercising at different levels at any time in their lives. If you are unsure about how much and what sort of exercise you should do, it's a good idea to pay a visit to your doctor for advice, especially if you have any medical conditions or you haven't taken much exercise since you left school.

Exercise programmes are available for everyone – pregnant women, seniors and disabled people alike. Age-related symptoms are often alleviated by increased mobility and activity and many recreation facilities have specialized classes for people who may have mobility problems or

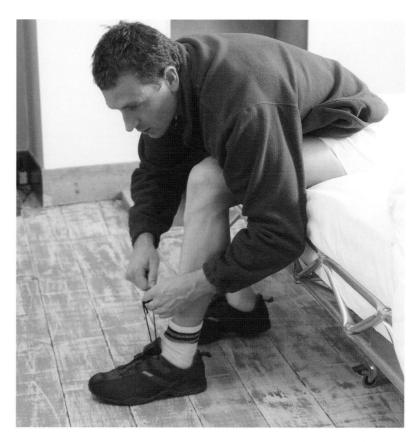

special needs. It is well worth visiting your local gym or recreation facility and talking to a trained professional about the options available and their suitability to your particular needs. Fitness professionals are extremely welcoming and motivating to everyone who is interested in increasing their fitness levels and the chances are that they will give you the utmost support to help you achieve your goals.

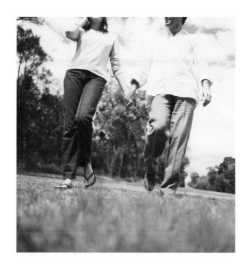

ABOVE | Running is a great way to get fit and increase your stamina and, apart from the cost of a pair of good, supportive running shoes, it's completely free.

BELOW LEFT | There are many kinds of exercise you can try, whatever your age. Just taking a walk in the open air together whenever you can will keep you in shape.

yoga and pilates

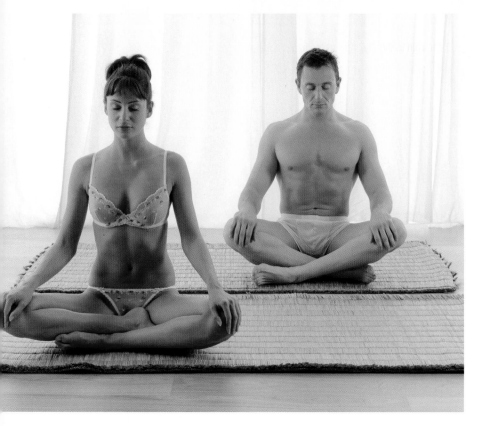

ABOVE | Practising yoga increases suppleness and flexibility, which makes for great sex. PC exercises contract the anal muscles, PC muscle and navel into the body, increasing energy, while strengthening other muscles in the area.

A GREAT SEX LIFE is dependent on good health, and one aspect of keeping well is keeping fit. You will benefit by keeping your heart and lungs strong and your muscles toned. There are certain exercises that women in particular need to do to keep themselves sexually fit. As they get older, muscles become flabbier if they are not worked and when women hit the menopause, the muscles begin to weaken even more. This also applies to the PC (puboccygeus) muscle. This is the pelvic floor muscle that runs between the legs from the anus to the genitals in both men and women and is the muscle that contracts at a rate of just under once a second during orgasm. If a man has a strong PC muscle, it will help him control the timing of his orgasm.

Yoga and pilates are beneficial and holistic forms of exercise for both men and women. It is a good idea to start any new exercise regime by attending a class before you try to do it by yourself.

Find one that suits you and try to go with your partner at least once a week. Once you have learned some of the positions, you can practise at home with the aid of a book or a video. Working on some of the postures, like hip openers, will help you to achieve more complex sexual positions that you thought you would never do again.

pelvic tilt

This is a marvellous exercise to flatten your stomach muscles and keep you feeling good about your body. Lie on your back, placing your hands on your pelvis with the fingertips on the pubic bone and the pads of your hands resting on the pelvic bones. Breathe in and lengthen through the top of your head. Breathe out and draw up the pelvic floor muscles and pull the lower abdominals back towards the spine, hollowing out your lower stomach (this is referred to as zip up and hollow, which is a requirement for almost all the exercises). Keep your tailbone on the floor lengthening away and do not push into the spine or tuck under the pelvis. You are in neutral position. Breathe in and then relax.

Try this again, with your legs flat on the floor. Lie on your back, lengthening your spine through your head. Your legs should be shoulder-width apart and totally relaxed. Your arms should be by your side with palms facing up. Breathe in to prepare, breathe out and zip up and hollow from the pelvic floor. The tailbone should be on the floor lengthening away. Breathe in and relax.

scissors

Lie on a mat, bend your knees to your chest and hold your right leg behind the thigh. Breathe in to prepare. Breathe out and zip up and hollow. Breathe in and straighten both legs in the air, pointing the toes. Breathe out, lengthen and lower the left leg, stopping just above the floor. Breathe in and raise the leg as straight as possible. Breathe out and change legs, crossing over like scissors.

the bridge

Begin by lying on your back with your knees bent and your feet flat on the floor close to your body and parallel to each other. Rest your arms alongside your body with your palms facing down. As you exhale, rotate your pelvis back and push the small of your back into the floor. As you inhale, lift your back off the floor, vertebra by vertebra, starting at the tailbone. Hold the pose for 15 to 30 seconds, or until you feel discomfort. Bring your spine back down to the floor in the same way, beginning with your upper back and stretching your spine towards your heels.

wall slide

The aim of this exercise is to lengthen the base of the spine without over-tilting the pelvis or tucking it under too far. At the same time it will strengthen the thigh muscles and stretch the Achilles tendon. Stand with your back against the wall and your feet hip-width apart and parallel, 15cm/6in from the wall. Place hands on hips or by your side. Lean back against the wall and breathe in, lengthening through the spine. Breathe out, pull up the pelvic floor and draw your lower abdominals back to the spine. Slide about 30cm/12in down the wall. Breathe in as you slide up. Repeat eight times.

the full hundred

Lie on the floor, or a comfortable mat or rug, with your knees bent and feet flat on the floor. Your arms should be by your side, palms down. Breathe in and prepare. Breathe out, zip up and hollow. Tuck the chin in slightly and curl the upper body off the floor, at the same time straightening one leg into the air. Reach through the fingertips, lengthening the shoulder blades down the back. Turn out your legs from the hips and flex the feet, lengthening through the heels, so you feel the stretch on the inside of your legs. Squeeze your inner thighs together and engage the pelvic floor. Breathe in for a count of five beats of the arms, then breathe out for five beats, moving the arms as if you were patting the floor. Continue for 100 beats then repeat with the other leg. For beginners, release the head and rest it on the floor.

the half hundred

This is a slightly more advanced version. Breathe in and prepare, breathe out, zip up and hollow. Tuck in the chin slightly and curl the upper body off the floor, or rest your head on the floor. This time bend both knees at the same time while you repeat the movements above. Keep this up regularly, and you will feel an improvement very quickly.

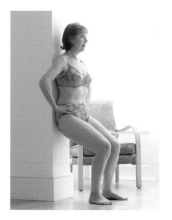

ABOVE | The wall slide will strengthen your legs and stomach muscles.

BELOW LEFT | The full hundred, with straight legs.

BELOW RIGHT | The half hundred, with knees bent.

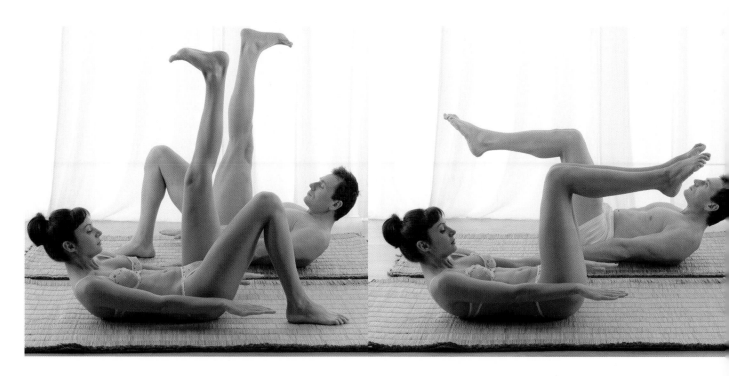

contraception and safer sex

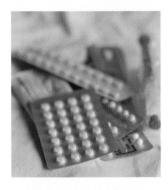

ABOVE | As well as the female pill, new male contraceptives are under development in the form of a transdermal gel and patch that rely on MENT™ (7a-methyl-19-nortestosterone), a synthetic steroid that resembles testosterone but lacks the unwanted side effect of an enlarged prostate.

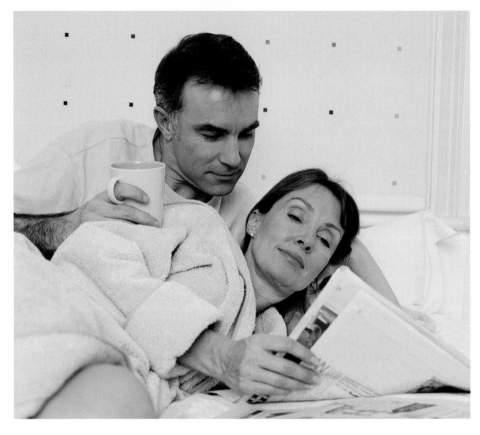

sterilization

Male and female sterilization are permanent methods of contraception that are 99 per cent effective. In female sterilization the fallopian tubes are either clipped, ringed or heat-treated to seal them. This prevents the sperm from meeting the egg. Male sterilization seals the tubes that carry the sperm to the penis from the testicles. Unlike female sterilization, vasectomy takes a while to work and it is necessary to use other contraceptives until the doctor gives the all clear.

WHEN DECIDING ON suitable contraception methods there are a several factors to be considered: age, lifestyle, health, whether you have children, and whether you may want to have children in the future. No contraceptive is 100 per cent effective. For extra peace of mind you can always use more than one product – such as the contraceptive pill combined with condoms.

hormonal methods

The contraceptive pill is hormone-controlled contraception. The combined pill combines the two hormones oestrogen and progesterone to prevent the monthly release of an egg. If taken correctly, it is 99 per cent effective, but may not be suitable for women who have high blood pressure, circulatory disease or diabetes. The progesterone-only pill, or minipill, causes cervical mucus to form a thick barrier which prevents sperm from entering the

uterus; it also makes the uterine lining thinner to prevent fertilized eggs from attaching to the wall. It is advised for breastfeeding mothers, older women and smokers. It is 98 per cent effective.

For longer acting contraception, an injection is now available which is 99 per cent effective. It slowly releases progesterone, preventing ovulation. Each injection lasts for 8–12 weeks. Side effects can include continual menstruation or none at all.

Implanon is a progesterone implant, which acts in a similar way by releasing progesterone into the body. It is 99 per cent effective and lasts for three years, but can lead to irregular periods or even cause them to stop altogether.

barrier methods

If used properly, condoms are 94–98 per cent effective and protect against STIs such as HIV and AIDS. They should be placed on as soon as the penis is erect because it can drip semen before ejaculation and men must withdraw as soon as they ejaculate. Female condoms are made of thin polyurethane plastic. They fit inside the vagina and prevent sperm from entering. If used correctly, they are 95 per cent effective.

The diaphragm or cap is another method of barrier contraceptive that is 92–96 per cent effective. It is a rubber dome that fits over the woman's cervix to prevent sperm from entering the uterus. It must be used in conjunction with spermicidal jelly or pessaries and should stay in place for six hours after sex.

intrauterine methods

The IUD is a T-shaped plastic device that works by stopping the sperm from reaching the egg and preventing the egg from implanting in the uterus. IUDs can make periods heavier and more painful and are not suitable for women who have more than one sexual partner as they can increase the risk of infection. Some women's bodies have rejected – and ejected – IUDs, but they have often not realized it until they became pregnant. The IUS works in a similar way to the IUD, but contains the hormones progesterone and oestrogen, which are gradually released into the body. This system can reduce heavy periods and period pains and is over 99 per cent effective. Gynefix has a more flexible frame. It is composed of a row of copper beads, which bend to fit snugly inside the uterus, and has

a fine nylon thread attaching it to the uterine wall, so it is more secure and less likely to be expelled. It can also assist in relieving heavy and painful periods and has been shown to be more than 99 per cent effective as a contraceptive. All three devices can remain inside a woman for up to five years and doctors teach women how to check for the threads of their IUDs or IUSs to make sure that they are still in place. This is critical and all women fitted with such devices should check regularly.

natural methods

Using natural methods of contraception involves identifying the fertile days of the woman's menstrual cycle and abstaining from sex during these days. The fertile time is the time when she is ovulating. Although the egg will only live for about 24 hours, sperm in a woman's body can survive for much longer, so sex a week before ovulation can still result in pregnancy.

Noting the different signs of ovulation can be done by either using a hormone-testing kit, the temperature method or noting dates and cervical secretions. Many women prefer natural methods as there are no side effects or chemicals involved. Success relies not only on the organization and discipline of the couple but also may be affected by age, stress, illness, hormonal treatments, irregular periods and the menopause. Natural methods claim to be 94–98 per cent effective, as long as the instructions are carefully implemented.

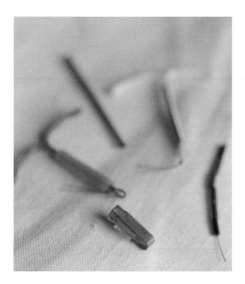

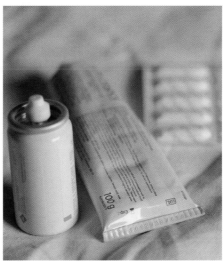

FAR LEFT | IUDs can last for 5–10 years and are a good long-term contraceptive.

LEFT | A variety of spermicides are available in cream or pessary form.

changing needs

THERE ARE VARIOUS FORMS OF CONTRACEPTION for different needs and different times of life. While your body changes throughout your life, one thing is certain: if you are fertile and sexually active, and don't want babies, you need to use some form of contraception. Your doctor, gynaecologist or family planning advisor will be able to give you the best advice for your age and health. Many of the more popular contraceptives are just not suitable for some people. The pill, for example, is not good for smokers. The coil (IUD) is not an ideal contraceptive for women who have not yet given birth and the condom is not 100 per cent reliable. In fact, no form of contraception is 100 per cent reliable, so it is best to have another strategy just in case. For example, if you are on the pill, you should consider using condoms as well.

Couples should decide together about contraception. It is generally women who take responsibility – they are the ones who risk getting pregnant, and they also have a bigger choice of contraception; men are mostly limited to the condom or to having a vasectomy. (The male pill hasn't proved to be a great success.)

Male vasectomy is less risky than female sterilization. It is a big step, so it is wise to think about it very carefully and to consider all the implications. If you do go ahead, and subsequently start another relationship, don't forget that a vasectomy will not protect you from sexually transmitted infections.

When you reach the menopause, don't be fooled into thinking that you cannot conceive. Even if your periods are irregular, you must continue to use contraception until a year after your last period and until you are finally given the all clear, through a hormone test.

infertility

As people age, fertility levels change, most notably in women. Women reach the menopause in midlife, resulting in an inability to have any

BELOW | Couples need to offer mutual support and discuss changing contraceptive needs together.

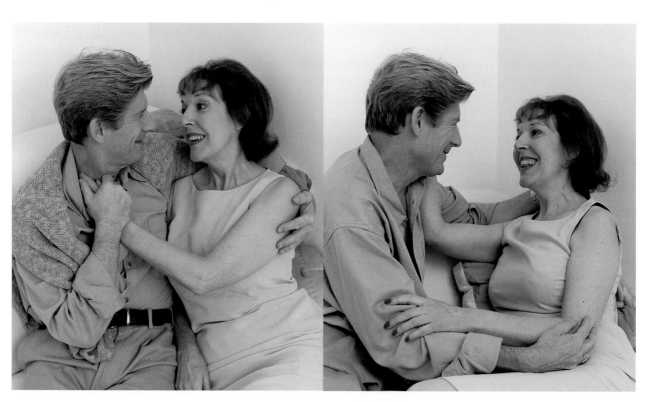

more children. Although men are normally able to father children throughout their lives, their fertility can be affected by problems such as low sperm count or age-related impotence and erectile difficulties. A young, fertile, healthy couple has an approximately one in four chance of conceiving a baby with each cycle. Once the woman reaches the age of 35, the odds of conceiving become greatly reduced, to 10 per cent each cycle. At this stage, some couples seek medical assistance in the form of hormone treatment or in-vitro fertilization (IVF).

Couples trying for a baby need to be in tune with the woman's menstrual cycle, so that they are aware of when she is at her most fertile. The ovaries release an egg each month in the middle of the menstrual cycle, around the 14th day. A woman can be fertile for a few days before and 24 hours after she ovulates. Sperm has a better chance of reaching the egg, however, if it is ejaculated into the vagina 24 hours before the egg is released, as sperm can stay alive in the woman's body for two to three days.

During ovulation, the woman may notice that her mucus discharge is thinner and stringier than at other times. Another way of knowing when the egg is released is by using an ovulation tester kit that detects hormonal changes. An alternative method is to chart changes in the woman's body temperature using a basal body temperature thermometer. When the woman ovulates, her temperature rises by about 0.2 to 0.6 degrees and remains higher until her next period. When she becomes pregnant, her body maintains this increased temperature.

ivf

In-vitro fertilization is a procedure that stimulates egg production through drug and hormone therapy. The growth of ovarian follicles is checked by ultrasound and when the follicles reach the correct size, hormones are administered to cause the eggs to be released. The eggs are harvested using a fine needle guided by an ultrasound image. The eggs are then incubated at body temperature for four to six hours before sperm is added. The fertilized

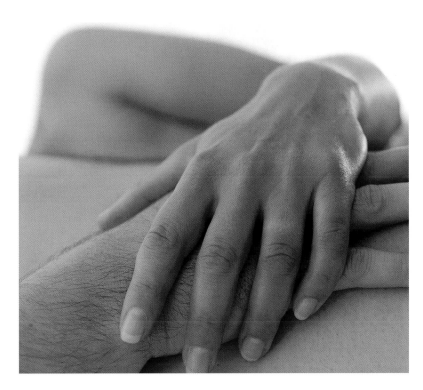

eggs are kept in a culture medium for around two days, before one or more is implanted in the woman's uterus using a fine needle. At present, this procedure is still fraught with difficulties and only around 10 per cent of attempts are successful, making it the least successful method of conceiving artificially. It is often seen as a last resort, not just because of its failure rate, but also because it is fairly unpleasant to undergo.

Another artificial method is used for couples where the man has a low sperm count. This involves injecting a single sperm directly into the ovary via a fine needle. This method has been highly criticized, as there is some evidence that it may increase the likelihood of birth defects. It is also suggested that it interferes with the natural selection process by which only the fittest sperm reach the egg, and that sperm taken from men with a very low sperm count may contain a genetic mutation that could pass on male infertility to future generations.

IVF is expensive, both financially and in terms of the couple's emotions. Couples considering IVF are required to consult a professional expert beforehand to go through their options and get all the counselling that they will need.

ABOVE | A course of IVF treatment can be an ordeal emotionally, physically and financially, so make sure you go into it together.

fertile ground

Many factors affect the fertility of both men and women. Overeating, smoking, stress and drugs all have a negative effect on sperm production. The correction of mineral deficiencies and eating organic produce are thought by some to improve libido and fertility by up to about 86 per cent.

sexual problems

AT SOME POINT DURING YOUR LIFE, your sexual activity is likely to be interrupted and temporarily halted. This could either be as a result of physical illness, such as heart problems or major surgery, or the outcome of psychological challenges involving bereavement, breakdown of a relationship or depression, or a combination. It is crucial to get to the bottom of the problem by discussing it with your partner, a doctor or a sex therapist.

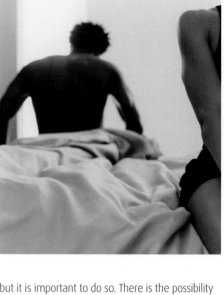

men's problems

Men can suffer from performance problems at any time during their life, either in the form of premature ejaculation, erectile dysfunction or an inability to ejaculate. A vicious circle can occur if, following an isolated incident of impotence, a man is so worried the next time he makes love that it occurs again. In this situation a period of sexual abstinence until his normal sex drive reasserts itself will usually solve the problem. Many men find it difficult to talk about their health problems, but it is important to do so. There is the possibility of sildenafil, the "wonder pill" that increases the penis's ability to achieve and maintain an erection once a man is sexually aroused. Every man who is thinking of taking such drugs should have a medical check-up first, as a number of serious side effects have been reported.

BELOW AND RIGHT |
A temporary loss of libido is very common in long-term relationships. It can be devastating for both partners when it happens, whether caused by emotional or physical problems. However, with the right help, it is usually overcome.

women's problems

There are several problems that are common amongst women. Pain while having sex may have physical or psychological causes. It can simply be the result of inadequate lubrication, especially with older women. In that case, the remedy is simple — avail yourself of the exotic, flavoured gels available from sex shops. If the pain is deep, then it could result from infection or cysts and you should consult your doctor. Psychological problems may vary in severity. Many can be resolved with the help of an understanding partner and a loving touch that stops short of penetration until the woman feels ready. More severe or long-term problems will require professional help. As with men, women's sex lives will be affected by illnesses such as diabetes, heart disease or high blood pressure. Your doctor will able to advise you and help you to resume a normal sex life.

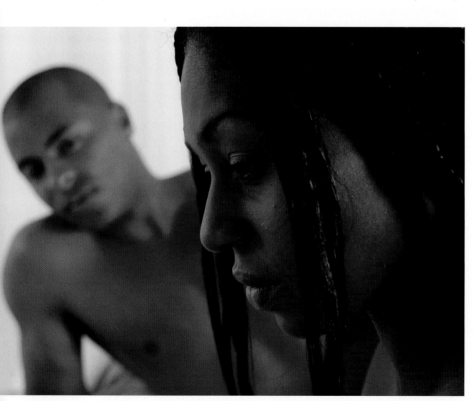

loss of libido

The loss of libido can affect both men and women and the causes are often very common things, such as stress, depression, physical illness, overwork or relationship problems. In men, it is a fast-growing problem, owing in part to the strain of today's competitive workplace. Many antidepressants, such as Prozac, are known to have a negative effect on sexual desire. It is important to continue any medication until you have consulted your doctor, who will be able to advise you and offer a possible alternative. Sometimes lack of libido is just a symptom of another problem that can be investigated.

painful intercourse

Sexual intercourse should not be painful, but a large number of women suffer for some time before seeking help. Painful intercourse, or dyspareunia, can have a variety of causes from vaginismus (involuntary spasms of the vaginal walls) to lack of lubrication or arousal. The main thing is to take action, not to suffer in silence, as the solution may be simpler than you think.

premature ejaculation

Many men experience premature ejaculation at some point, but you can train yourself to control your orgasm. Begin by masturbating and bring yourself close to ejaculation. Stop, relax and start again. Repeat until you can't control the orgasm any further. The point is to learn when you are about to climax, so the more you practise, the more you are likely to be able to delay your orgasm to the point at which you want to come. Once you have accomplished this, experiment with your partner. While she is masturbating you, ask her to stop when you are about to ejaculate. Again, stop, relax and start again.

The squeeze technique is another way of achieving the same result. Either you or your partner can squeeze the tip of your penis just before climax. The squeeze forces the blood out of the penis and reduces the erection. Something else which might help is wearing a condom as prophylactics reduce sexual sensation during sex.

delayed ejaculation

This occurs in some men who find it difficult to reach orgasm even though they may want to and are receiving the necessary stimulation. The reason it happens is either physiological – due to diseases such as diabetes or prostatic disease, or certain types of drug therapy – or psychological where some men may have become repressed or inhibited. Psychosexual therapy can teach men how to overcome the inhibitory behaviour or fears that have become conditioned in them.

retrograde ejaculation

This occurs when men feel the sensation of ejaculation and orgasm but no fluid comes out. Semen is expelled from the testicles but instead of following the contractions and going through the urethra, it travels back into the bladder via the bladder neck. This is relatively common in men who have undergone prostatectomy. Other reasons for its occurrence are disruption of the nervous system caused by spinal cord injury, diabetes, multiple sclerosis and some prescription medications.

erectile dysfunction

During adolescence, young men are frequently embarrassed by how readily an erection occurs. With increasing age it doesn't happen so often, it isn't so firm and it doesn't last so long. By the time this happens, most men should be mature enough to explore other options, from oral sex to a simple change of position. Alcohol can be the culprit when the spirit is willing but the flesh is weak. Surprisingly, erectile problems as a result of drinking too much – sometimes known as brewer's droop – affect young men more frequently than older men.

Impotence may be caused by a neurological disorder, where nerve signals are interrupted; problems with the blood flow; hormonal deficiency; diabetes or infection. Not surprisingly, perhaps, men are reluctant to seek help, although many treatments are available. One of the most widely known is Viagra (sildenafil), although this is only effective for one-third of users. Other treatments include vacuum pumps used with a constricting ring, penile implants and urethral injections.

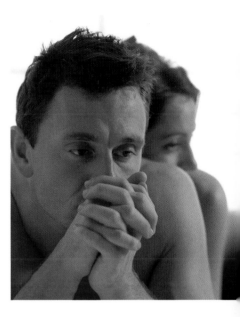

ABOVE | Ejaculation problems can be terribly frustrating but it is important to maintain a perspective on the situation. Sensitivity combined with humour can help, while removing the emphasis from penetration and concentrating on foreplay can divert attention away from the problem and restore confidence.

glossary

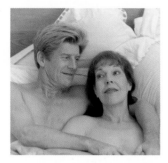

anal Relating to the anus, as in anal sex.

aphrodisiac An experience or substance that stimulates or enhances sexual desire.

blow job Oral sex done on a man; fellatio.

bondage Sexual arousal by physical restrictions, such as handcuffs and rope restraints.

CAT Coital Alignment Technique – an intercourse technique where you roll rather than thrust.

cervical cap Birth control device that covers the cervix and acts as a barrier to prevent the sperm from entering.

chakras Described in Tantric sex. These are the seven points in individuals, which are believed to regulate different types of energy.

clitoris The only organ in the human body whose sole function is pleasure.

condom A latex sheath that fits over the penis is the most common form of barrier contraception.

diaphragm Contraceptive barrier method which holds spermicidal jelly against the cervical opening.

dildo Penis-shaped object, which can be inserted into the vagina or anus for sexual stimulation.

ejaculate The white fluid which usually accompanies male orgasm.

impotence When a man is unable to get an erection on a regular basis.

IUD Formerly known as the coil, a device fitted into the uterus that prevents conception by stopping the egg implanting in the uterus wall.

Kama Sutra An Indian classical book on the technique and art of love and lovemaking.

kundalini Derived from the Sanskrit word "kundal" meaning coiled up, which is normally represented as a coiled or sleeping serpent in Vedic and Tantric texts.

libido The desire that drives us to have a sexual relationship with another person.

lingham Sanskrit for penis.

maithuna A skill men use to suppress their orgasm in Tantric sex.

masturbation Stimulating your own genitals to achieve sexual gratification.

merkin A wig made specifically for the pubic region, held on with glue.

morning after pill Emergency contraception that can be used up to 72 hours after unprotected sex.

orgasm The sensations that ripple through your body at the climax of sexual excitement.

pelvic tilt An exercise to keep the muscles of the pelvis in trim.

pessaries Spermicides in the form of small bullets which are inserted into the vagina.

Pilates A gentle form of exercise for the body inspired by Joseph Pilates.

pranayama A breathing technique in yoga.

prostate The gland that is responsible for a portion of the male ejaculate, it contracts seconds before orgasm. Located on the floor of the rectum.

puboccygeus (PC) muscle This holds the pelvic floor together.

rimming Kissing and licking the anus.

Sanskrit The ancient Indo-European literary language of India.

scissors A Pilates-based exercise holding the legs in the air and making a scissor action.

soixante-neuf (69) Where a couple perform oral sex on each other simultaneously.

spermicide A cream, gel or pessary that will kill sperm on contact, often added to condoms.

STI Sexually transmitted infection. Also known as STD (sexually transmitted disease).

swinging Husband-and-wife-swapping, often involving group sex or specific parties where couples swap and have sex with other partners.

Tantra A number of Hindu and Buddhist writings giving religious teaching and ritual instructions.

vibrator An electrical vibrating device used most commonly by women for masturbation. Can be used vaginally or anally.

voyeurism A fetish involving individuals achieving sexual stimulation from watching other people undress or have sex.

yoni The Sanskrit word for a woman's vulva, a term often used in Tantra.

useful addresses & acknowledgements

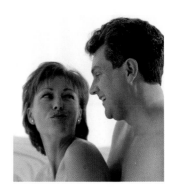

American Counseling Association

5999 Stevenson Avenue, Alexandria, Virginia 22304

(800) 347–6647

www.counseling.org

British Association for Sexual and Relationship Therapy (BASRT)

National charity with a list of therapists.

PO Box 13686, London SW20 92H

020 8543 2707

www.basrt.org.uk

fpa (formerly the Family Planning Association)

50 Featherstone Street, London EC1Y 8QU

Helpline: 0845 122 8690

www.fpa.org.uk

Marie Stopes International

Sexual and reproductive health information.

www.mariestopes.org.uk

www.mariestopes.org.au

National AIDS Helpline

0800 567123 (24 hours)

Outsiders Sex and Disability Helpline

Dr Tuppy Owen, BCM Box Lovely,

London WC1N 3XX

Helpline: 0707 499 3527

www.outsiders.org.uk

Relate – the relationship people

The UK's largest and most experienced relationship support organization.

Herbert Gray College, Little Church Street, Rugby, Warwickshire CV21 3AP

0845 456 1310

www.relate.org.uk

Relationships Australia

PO Box 313, Curtin ACT 2605

02 6285 4466

relationships.com.au

I would like to say a special thank you to my two colleagues: firstly Clare Spurrell, a budding writer and adventurer who has contributed greatly to the book both in research and editorially, and secondly Tessa Swithinbank, who is a writer and very close friend who has also been a great support and contributor to this book. I would also like to thank Ruth Thomson, Tannis Taylor, Jonathan Hart, Emily Dubberley from cliterati.co.uk, Lynn Warner, Robert Page from *The Lovers' Guide*, Trilby Fairfax, Simon Parritt from SPOD, Robert and Lynn Watson from Dateable, Dr Jane Roy from Relate and all my other pals who were kind enough to talk to me about their sex lives and fantasies, my editor, Katy Bevan and copy editor Sarah Brown, the photographer John Freeman, his assistant Alex Dow, and make–up artist Bettina Graham. And for using their bodies to illustrate the text, Katy and Nathan, Helen and Armani, Tino and Jennifer, Steve and Barbara, Jessica and Kitt, and Justin and Abigail. Marie Stopes provided the items for contraception. Sh! Women's Erotic Emporium, Coco de Mer and

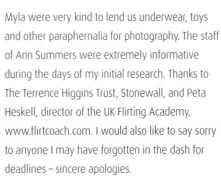

Myla were very kind to lend us underwear, toys and other paraphernalia for photography. The staff of Ann Summers were extremely informative during the days of my initial research. Thanks to The Terrence Higgins Trust, Stonewall, and Peta Heskell, director of the UK Flirting Academy, www.flirtcoach.com. I would also like to say sorry to anyone I may have forgotten in the dash for deadlines – sincere apologies.

Finally I would like to dedicate this book to all of the men in my life who in their own way have helped me write this book: my father and greatest supporter, Jessel, followed by my many relatives, and much–loved friends past and present: Dominic, Stuart, John, Gil, Charlie, Robert, Roger (who insisted that I mention him) and to B.K. my inspiration.

Thanks to the following for the loan of gorgeous props for photography:
The Cloth Shop, **Coco de Mer, Ganesha London, Myla, Sh!, The White Company.**

index

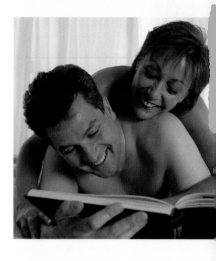